MRCS CORE MODULES: MCQs & EMQs

Andrew Williams MBBS BSc FRCS
Surgical Registrar
Bromley Hospital, Bromley, Kent

Tom Hennigan MBBS FRCS
Colorectal and laparoscopic surgeon
Bromley Hospital, Bromley, Kent

Christopher L H Chan BSc FRCS
Specialist Registrar in General Surgery
St. Thomas' Hospital, London

Lindsey Barker BSc MB ChB FRCS
Specialist Registrar in General Surgery
Kent and Canterbury Hospitals NHS Trust,
Canterbury, Kent

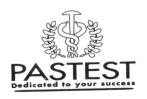

PASTEST
Dedicated to your success

© 1999 PASTEST
Egerton Court
Parkgate Estate
Knutsford
Cheshire WA16 8DX

Telephone: 01565 755226

First published 1999

ISBN: 1 901198 09X

A catalogue record for this book is available from the British Library.

The information contained within this book was obtained by the authors from reliable sources. However, while every effort has been made to ensure its accuracy, no responsibilty for loss, damage or injury occasioned to any person acting or refraining from action as a result of information contained herein can be accepted by the publishers or authors.

PasTest Revision Books and Intensive Courses
PasTest has been established in the field of postgraduate medical education since 1972, providing revision books and intensive study courses for doctors preparing for their professional examinations.
Books and courses are available for the following specialties:
MRCP Part 1 and Part 2 (General Medicine and Paediatrics), MRCOG, DRCOG, MRCGP, DCH, FRCA, FRCS, PLAB.
For further details contact:

**PasTest, Freepost, Knutsford, Cheshire WA16 7BR
Tel: 01565 755226   Fax: 01565 650264**

Text prepared by Breeze Limited, Manchester.
Printed and bound by Biddles Ltd, Guildford and Kings Lynn.

CONTENTS

MCQ EXAMINATION TECHNIQUE

Before sitting an MCQ examination, you will need to know how many questions are likely to be on the paper and how long you will be given to complete it. Thus you will be able to assess the approximate amount of time that can be spent on each question. The time allotted for each of the written papers is **two hours**. Different questions are used each time, therefore subject composition is variable from exam to exam. There are approximately 45 MCQs questions and around 20 EMQs, depending upon the number of responses required.

Pacing yourself accurately during the examination to finish on time, or with time to spare, is essential. You must also decide on your own personal strategy for approaching the paper. You may decide to read quickly through the paper before picking up your pen, or to work slowly through the paper answering everything that you are certain of and leaving anything you wish to come back to.

There are two common mistakes which cause good candidates to fail the MRCS written examinations. These are neglecting to read the directions and questions carefully enough and failing to fill in the computer answer card properly. You must read the instructions to candidates at the beginning of each section of the paper to ensure that you complete the answer sheet correctly. You must also ensure that you read the question (both stem and items) carefully. Regard each item as being independent of every other item, each referring to a specific quantum of knowledge. The item (or the stem and the item taken together) make up a statement as "True" or "False". The number of stems will vary for each question. For this reason, a mark will not necessarily be required for each column of the answer sheet. For every correct answer you will gain a mark (+1). For the MRCS (London) examination, marks will not be deducted for a wrong answer. Equally, you will not gain a mark if you mark both true and false.

You must also decide on a strategy to follow with regard to marking your answers. The answer sheet is read by an automatic document reader, which transfers the information it reads to a computer. It is critical that the answer sheet is filled in clearly and accurately using the pencils provided. Failure to fill in your name and your examination correctly could result in the rejection of your paper.

Some candidates mark their answers directly onto the computer sheet as they go through the question, others prefer to make a note of their answers on the question paper, and reserve time at the end to transfer their answers onto the computer sheet. If you choose the first method, there is a chance that you may decide to change your answer after a second reading. If you do change your answer on the computer sheet, you must ensure that your original is thoroughly erased. If you choose the second method, make sure that you allow enough time to transfer your answers methodically onto the computer sheet, as rushing at this stage could introduce some costly mistakes. You will find it less confusing if you transfer your marks after you have completed each section of the examination.

MCQ Examination Technique

You must ensure that you have left sufficient time to transfer your marks from the question paper to the answer sheet. You should also be aware that no additional time will be given at the end of the examination to allow you to transfer your marks.

If you find that you have time left at the end of the examination, there can be a temptation to re-read your answers time and time again, so that even those that seemed straightforward will start to look less convincing. In this situation, first thoughts are usually the best, don't alter your initial answers unless you are sure. Don't be afraid to leave the examination room once you are satisfied with your answers.

To guess or not to guess

Tests carried out at PasTest's MRCS intensive revision courses have proved that by far the majority of candidates can improve their marks by making sensible guesses.

The MRCS exams in England are not negatively marked[1]. For this reason you should answer every question as you have nothing to lose. If you do not know the answer to a question, you should make an educated guess - you may well get the answer right and gain a mark.

If you feel that you need to spend more time puzzling over a question, leave it and, if you have time, return to it. Make sure you have collected all the marks you can before you come back to any difficult questions.

Final advice

Multiple choice questions are not designed to trick you or confuse you, they are designed to test your knowledge of medicine. Accept each question at its face value, do not look for hidden meanings or catches.

The aim of this book is to enable you to evaluate your level of knowledge by working through the questions in each section. By marking clearly all of the answers that you got wrong or declined to answer, you can then refresh your memory with the explanations given here or read up on specific topics in depth using a textbook.

Working through the questions in this book will help you to identify your weak subject areas. Using books and lectures, you must work out your own personal profile of strengths and weaknesses and plan your revision accordingly. In the last few weeks before the exam it will be important for you to avoid minor unimportant areas and concentrate on the most important subject areas covered in the exam.

---

[1] The AFRCS examinations in Scotland are currently negatively marked.

ABBREVIATIONS

ADH	Anti-diuretic hormone	HCC	Hydrocholecalciferol
AFP	Alpha-fetoprotein	HLA	Human leucocyte antigen
AIDS	Acquired immune deficiency syndrome	ICP	Intra-cranial pressure
APTT	Activated partial thromboplastin time	INR	International normalised ratio
		IPPV	Intermittent positive pressure ventilation
ARDS	Acute respiratory distress syndrome	IVU	Intravenous urogram
ASA	American Society of Anaesthesiologists	JVP	Jugular venous pressure
		LH	Luteinising hormone
AV	Atrio-ventricular	LMWH	Low molecular weight heparin
BMI	Body mass index	MCV	Mean corpuscular volume
BP	Blood pressure	MEN	Multiple endocrine neoplasia
CEA	Carcinoembryonic antigen	MI	Myocardial infarction
CMF	Cyclophosphamide, methotrexate, 5-fluorouracil	MNCG	Multi-nodular colloid goitre
		MRI	Magnetic resonance imaging
CMV	Cytomegalovirus	MRSA	Methicillin-resistant *Staphylococcus aureus*
COPD	Chronic obstructive pulmonary disease	MSU	Midstream urine
CPAP	Continuous positive airway pressure	NdYAG	Neodymium yttrium aluminium garnet
CSF	Cerebro spinal fluid	NG	Naso-gastric
CT	Computerised tomography	NSAID	Non-steroidal anti-inflammatory drugs
CVP	Central venous pressure		
CVS	Cardiovascular system	PAN	Polyarteritis nodosa
DCIS	Ductal carcinoma in situ	PCA	Patient controlled analgesia
DSA	Digital subtraction angiography	PE	Pulmonary embolism
DU	Duodenal ulcer	PEEP	Positive end expiratory pressure
DVT	Deep vein thrombosis	PHPT	Primary hyperparathyroidism
ECG	Electrocardiograph	PSA	Prostatic specific antigen
EPL	Extensor pollicis longus	PTH	Parathyroid hormone
ESWL	Extracorporeal shock wave lithotripsy	RA	Rheumatoid arthritis
		RBC	Red blood cell
ET	Endotracheal	SAH	Subarachnoid haemorrhage
FAP	Familial adenomatous polyposis	SCD	Sickle cell disease
FDPs	Fibrinogen degradation products	SLE	Systemic lupus erythematosus
FEV_1	Forced expiratory volume in one second	TCC	Transitional cell carcinoma
		TED	Thromboembolism deterrent
FFP	Fresh frozen plasma	TENS	Transcutaneous electrical nerve stimulation
FNAC	Fine needle aspiration cytology		
FRC	Functional residual capacity	TIA	Transient ischaemic attack
FVC	Flow volume capacity	TNF	Tumour necrosis factor
GA	General anaesthesia	TPN	Total parenteral nutrition
GFR	Glomerular filtration rate	UC	Ulcerative colitis
GI	Gastro-intestinal	UICC	International union against cancer
GIT	Gastro-intestinal tract	UTIs	Urinary Tract Infections
GMCSF	Granulocyte macrophage colony stimulating factor	WBC	White blood cell
		WCC	White cell count
GORD	Gastro-oesophageal reflux disease	WR	Wasserman reaction

1.1 To be suitable for day surgery under general anaesthesia the patient

❑ A should have a friend or relative to stay with them on the first night
❑ B could be undergoing haemorrhoidectomy
❑ C may have a body mass index (BMI) of 34
❑ D could be undergoing a laparoscopic cholecystectomy
❑ E could be ASA grade 3
❑ F could have insulin-controlled diabetes mellitus
❑ G could be undergoing an axillary clearance for breast cancer

1.2 For procedures done in day surgery

❑ A premedication is required
❑ B spinal anaesthesia is a suitable technique
❑ C caudal block is a suitable technique
❑ D femoral nerve block is a suitable technique
❑ E drains should not be used

1.3 Co-amoxiclav

❑ A has activity against anaerobic organisms
❑ B is associated with cholestatic jaundice
❑ C may be used to treat MRSA
❑ D is active against penicillinase producing bacteria
❑ E is exclusively removed by first pass metabolism

1.4   *Clostridium tetani*

- ❏ A   may cause endotoxic shock
- ❏ B   affects the motor and sensory neurones of the central nervous system
- ❏ C   has an average incubation period of two weeks
- ❏ D   spreads through the wound
- ❏ E   is a Gram-positive bacillus with round terminal spores
- ❏ F   may cause gas gangrene

1.5   The following are associated with the acute response to injury:

- ❏ A   increased plasma catecholamines
- ❏ B   increased liver glycogen levels
- ❏ C   reduced insulin levels
- ❏ D   relative hypoglycaemia
- ❏ E   raised plasma fatty acids

1.6   *Bacteroides* species are

- ❏ A   non-sporing Gram-positive anaerobes
- ❏ B   uncommon in the female genital tract
- ❏ C   rarely found in the mouth
- ❏ D   sensitive to metronidazole
- ❏ E   resistant to gentamicin

1.7   The following are true of 'scrubbing up':

- ❏ A   hands become sterile
- ❏ B   the first scrub of the list is ineffective
- ❏ C   hot air dryers are a safe alternative to hand towels
- ❏ D   povidone-iodine is as effective as chlorhexidine
- ❏ E   it is unnecessary for dirty cases

1.8 Acute alcohol withdrawal

❑ A   can be readily anticipated
❑ B   is associated with abdominal wound dehiscence
❑ C   commonly causes convulsions
❑ D   may be treated with benzodiazepines
❑ E   should be treated by fluid restriction
❑ F   may cause acute renal failure
❑ G   may precipitate acute pancreatitis

1.9 Heat sensitive surgical equipment and materials may be sterilised by treatment with

❑ A   phenolic compounds
❑ B   buffered glutaraldehyde fluid
❑ C   ethylene oxide gas
❑ D   ethanol
❑ E   ionising radiation

1.10 Nutritional support

❑ A   is rarely indicated in multiple trauma
❑ B   can usually achieve a positive nitrogen balance in a septic patient
❑ C   should not be administered on a long-term basis by a fine bore nasogastric feeding tube
❑ D   should ideally be administered parenterally
❑ E   when used pre-operatively reduces post-operative complications after oesophagectomy
❑ F   prevents the development of ileus

1.11 Untreated pre-operative hypertension

- ❑ A is associated with increased incidence of stroke
- ❑ B is associated with increased incidence of perioperative MI
- ❑ C should be stabilised before elective surgery
- ❑ D predisposes to pulmonary embolism
- ❑ E may be controlled by sodium nitroprusside intra-operatively

1.12 *Escherichia coli*

- ❑ A is the commonest cause of nosocomial urinary tract sepsis
- ❑ B produces an exotoxin
- ❑ C is commonly resistant to gentamicin
- ❑ D may produce septic shock
- ❑ E frequently acquires plasmids leading to antibiotic resistance

1.13 Incidence of post-operative wound infection in abdominal surgery is increased with

- ❑ A extensive diathermy use
- ❑ B not wearing masks
- ❑ C inadequate haemostasis
- ❑ D well-controlled diabetes mellitus
- ❑ E steroid therapy
- ❑ F cyclosporin treatment

1.14 The following are true:

- ❑ A post amputation infection rates are reduced by 10% with pre-operative iodine baths
- ❑ B alcohol preparation of the skin is safe
- ❑ C alcohol based povidone-iodine is used for the perineum
- ❑ D chlorhexidine is a pink liquid
- ❑ E wound infection rates are reduced by the use of adhesive drapes

1.15   Human immunodeficiency virus (HIV)

❏ A   has been contracted by droplet aerosol created by orthopaedic power tools
❏ B   leads to a persistently elevated antigen titre
❏ C   most frequently leads to a reversal of the CD4/CD8 lymphocyte ratio
❏ D   has a transmission rate of about 1% following percutaneous exposure
❏ E   should be treated immediately with zidovudine following needle stick injury

1.16   A three day course of antibiotics is indicated in the following cases:

❏ A   excision of a normal appendix
❏ B   routine right hemicolectomy
❏ C   excision of perforated appendix
❏ D   Hartmann's procedure for a diverticular abscess
❏ E   drainage of a peri-anal abscess

1.17   In the assessment and preparation for general anaesthesia it is important to

❏ A   always note any family history of anaesthetic problems
❏ B   omit pre-operative oral hypoglycaemic agents
❏ C   omit pre-operative doses of bronchodilators
❏ D   routinely organise an ECG
❏ E   give all patients pre-medication to reduce anxiety

1.18   Opioids

❑   A   are not safe in the presence of asthma
❑   B   act mainly in the CNS
❑   C   such as diamorphine are partial μ agonists
❑   D   may be administered sublingually
❑   E   are metabolised in the liver into active and inactive products

1.19   In the assessment of a patient with COPD for surgery

❑   A   breathlessness at less than 50 metres is an indication for pulmonary function tests
❑   B $FEV_1 < 50\%$ of FVC is an indication for blood gas analysis
❑   C   post-operative course correlates well with resting $PaCO_2$ and PaO_2
❑   D   a $PaO_2 > 7.3$ kPa and a normal $PaCO_2$ indicates a poor prognosis
❑   E   cessation of smoking for > 1 month before operation has no post-operative benefit

1.20   Match the following with their description

❑   A   cyst
❑   B   papilloma
❑   C   plaque
❑   D   macule
❑   E   hamartoma

1.   elevated area
2.   flat lesion
3.   fluid filled tumour
4.   overgrowth of normal constituents
5.   overgrowth of epithelial tissue

1.21   The following metastasise:

❏   A   melanoma
❏   B   basal cell carcinoma
❏   C   squamous cell carcinoma
❏   D   turban tumour
❏   E   lentigo maligna

1.22   Patients with diabetes mellitus undergoing major surgery

❏   A   have an increased risk of wound complications
❏   B   have an increased bleeding tendency
❏   C   generally require less insulin during the procedure
❏   D   should be monitored by two hourly blood glucose
           measurements post-operatively
❏   E   should have the urine checked for ketones and glucose in the
           post-operative period

1.23   Patient controlled analgesia (PCA)

❏   A   requires post-operative monitoring with pulse oximetry
❏   B   rarely provides adequate analgesia
❏   C   usually involves a mixture of fentanyl and an anti-emetic
❏   D   possess a lock-out interval safety mechanism
❏   E   may cause respiratory depression

1.24   Tourniquets

❏   A   may be applied safely for up to three hours at a time
❏   B   should not be applied to a pressure exceeding 300 mmHg
❏   C   can cause focal demyelination of the peripheral nerve
❏   D   usually produce an axonotmesis
❏   E   are suitable for procedures under local anaesthesia

1.25 Plain bupivacaine

- ❏ A should not be used in a Bier's block
- ❏ B is more cardiotoxic than lignocaine
- ❏ C may exhibit tachyphylaxis
- ❏ D does not cross the placenta
- ❏ E has a maximum safe dose of 5 mg/kg

1.26 Face masks

- ❏ A should be worn by all members of staff in the operating theatre
- ❏ B contain filters made of polypropylene
- ❏ C may be re-used with safety
- ❏ D when wet lose their barrier qualities
- ❏ E protect the surgeon from airborne virus infection

1.27 Sterilisation by steam

- ❏ A does not kill heat-resistant spores
- ❏ B kills *Mycobacterium tuberculosis*
- ❏ C may be checked by Bowie Dick test
- ❏ D is suitable for fine surgical instruments
- ❏ E is performed under pressure at temperatures exceeding 200°C
- ❏ F is suitable for hernia repair mesh
- ❏ G is suitable for aortic knitted grafts
- ❏ H destroys MRSA

1.28 Pulse oximeters

- ❑ A only sense changes in arterial blood
- ❑ B are unaffected by carboxyhaemoglobin
- ❑ C are accurate to 0.5% above 90% oxygen saturation
- ❑ D may not indicate adequate ventilation
- ❑ E may not give accurate readings in hypovolaemic shock
- ❑ F are inaccurate under anaesthesia
- ❑ G produce false-negative results with chronic lung disease

1.29 Bipolar diathermy

- ❑ A involves the passage of low frequency alternating current through body tissue
- ❑ B requires a patient plate electrode
- ❑ C may have a cutting diathermy option
- ❑ D can be used in patients with pacemakers
- ❑ E should be avoided in circumcision

1.30 The NdYAG laser

- ❑ A has very little tissue penetration
- ❑ B is principally used for tattoo removal
- ❑ C has a role in palliation of oesophageal carcinoma
- ❑ D should be used in a designated Laser Controlled Area
- ❑ E user requires compulsory eye protection

1.31 Wound infection rates are reduced by the following:

- ❑ A peritoneal washout
- ❑ B the wearing of masks
- ❑ C shaving the operative site two days before surgery
- ❑ D prophylactic antibiotics
- ❑ E adhesive wound site dressings

1.32 Gram-negative bacilli

- ❑ A commonly cause meningitis
- ❑ B may be commensals in the gut
- ❑ C may cause food poisoning
- ❑ D occasionally infect serious burns
- ❑ E commonly cause pneumonia in COPD patients
- ❑ F are a common cause of liver abscesses

1.33 Commensal bacteria in different organs

- ❑ A cerebrospinal fluid
- ❑ B colon
- ❑ C upper respiratory tract
- ❑ D bile
- ❑ E bladder
- ❑ F stomach

For each of the above please select the single most appropriate option from below.

1. *Bacteroides fragilis*
2. *Gardnerella vaginalis*
3. *Streptococcus viridans*
4. *Neisseria meningitidis*
5. *Pneumocystis carinii*
6. *Staphylococcus aureus*
7. sterile

1.34   Wound infection rates are increased by the following:

❑   A   day case surgery
❑   B   diabetes mellitus
❑   C   poor surgical technique
❑   D   firm suturing
❑   E   the use of cutting diathermy

1.35   To minimise fire hazards in theatre

❑   A   rubber footwear should have a resistance of 1 MΩ
❑   B   electrical sockets should be sited above floor level
❑   C   a relative humidity of less than 60% is recommended
❑   D   cutting diathermy should only be used on rare occasions
❑   E   operating tables should be connected by high resistance to the floor

1.36   Day case surgery

❑   A   should allow junior surgeons to gain as much experience as possible
❑   B   is suitable for ASA grades I, II, III
❑   C   is ideally performed on operating lists with a mixture of day cases and inpatients
❑   D   leads to average inpatient costs rising

1.37   *Staphylococcus*

❑   A   is anaerobic
❑   B   is Gram-positive
❑   C   forms long strings
❑   D   *aureus* is coagulase positive
❑   E   may be grouped A to C

1.38 *Streptococcus*

☐ A causes cellulitis
☐ B *viridans* if found is usually pathological
☐ C *pneumoniae* form diplococci
☐ D may be α or β haemolytic
☐ E form clusters like bunches of grapes

1.39 Gram-positive rods

☐ A include *Clostridia* species
☐ B include *Enterococcus faecalis*
☐ C cause diarrhoea
☐ D may act via toxins
☐ E are all anaerobes

1.40 Adequate renal function is reflected by the following:

☐ A minimum urine output of 2 ml/kg/hour
☐ B urine osmolality in a fluid depleted patient of more than 460 mOsm/kg
☐ C creatinine of 200 mmol/l
☐ D normal MSU
☐ E diuresis of 10 ml/kg/hr on bolus dose of 20 mg frusemide
☐ F a normal blood pressure

1.41 T-tubes

☐ A should be removed after five days
☐ B are usually made from polyvinyl chloride
☐ C cause an intense fibrous reaction
☐ D are not affected by bile acids
☐ E are used less frequently with the advent of ERCP
☐ F should be brought out through the abdominal wound

1.42   Common features of an abscess include

❏   A   raised white blood count
❏   B   swinging pyrexia
❏   C   fluctuant swelling
❏   D   induration
❏   E   chronic discharge

1.43   Selection of drains for surgical procedures

❏   A   thyroidectomy
❏   B   primary inguinal hernia repair
❏   C   total hip replacement
❏   D   perforated appendix
❏   E   anterior resection
❏   F   perforated duodenal ulcer
❏   G   subphrenic abscess
❏   H   right hemicolectomy
❏   I   axillary clearance

For the procedures above select the single most appropriate option from below.

1.   sump
2.   corrugated
3.   suction
4.   tube drain
5.   none

1.44   Drug adverse reactions

❏   A   atenolol
❏   B   cisplatin
❏   C   glyceryl trinitrate
❏   D   NSAID

From each of the drugs above select the single most appropriate adverse effect from the list below.

1.   hypotension
2.   nephrotoxixity
3.   peptic ulceration
4.   bronchospasm
5.   bradycardia

1.45   Organisms and the infections they cause

❏   A   *H. influenzae*
❏   B   *E. coli*
❏   C   *Candida albicans*
❏   D   *Proteus*
❏   E   *Staph. aureus*
❏   F   *Strep. milleri*

For each of the organisms listed above select the single most appropriate infection from below.

1.   urinary tract infections
2.   oesophagitis
3.   endocarditis
4.   pneumonia
5.   wound infection
6.   liver abscess

1.46   In anaemic patients undergoing surgery

❑   A   the optimal pre-operative haemoglobin level is 12 g/dl
❑   B   a haemoglobin level of 10 g/dl is an indication for transfusion
❑   C   transfusion may be contraindicated in anaemia
❑   D   blood transfusion may increase the risk of recurrence of malignant tumours
❑   E   iron treatment should increase haemoglobin by 1 g/dl/month
❑   F   blood transfusion should be done the day prior to surgery

1.47   Disseminated intravascular coagulopathy (DIC) is

❑   A   associated with a platelet count 150 x 10^9/l
❑   B   associated with raised plasma fibrinogen degradation products
❑   C   associated with an INR greater than 1
❑   D   a contraindication to surgery
❑   E   an indication for Granulocyte Macrophage Colony Stimulating Factor administration
❑   F   associated with an increase in plasma fibrinogen

1.48   The long-term effects of steroids include

❑   A   bruising
❑   B   low mood
❑   C   hair loss
❑   D   better stress reaction to surgery
❑   E   weight gain
❑   F   thrombocytosis
❑   G   gingival hypertrophy
❑   H   osteopetrosis

1.49 **The following commonly improve outcome in a patient with chronic lung disease undergoing abdominal surgery:**

- ❑ A choice of incision
- ❑ B pre-operative ventilation
- ❑ C pre-operative chest physiotherapy
- ❑ D avoiding operating in the winter months
- ❑ E pre-operative antibiotics
- ❑ F stopping smoking two weeks prior to surgery
- ❑ G doxapram infusion
- ❑ H tracheostomy

1.50 **The following are used in the diagnosis of breast disease:**

- ❑ A ultrasound
- ❑ B contrast studies
- ❑ C magnetic resonance imaging
- ❑ D CT scanning
- ❑ E X-rays
- ❑ F duplex scanning
- ❑ G impedance tomography
- ❑ H radionuclide imaging

1.51 **Magnetic resonance imaging**

- ❑ A uses radio frequency waves
- ❑ B is poor for assessing the musculoskeletal system
- ❑ C cannot be used with contrast media
- ❑ D is safe after pacemaker insertion
- ❑ E is nearly always well tolerated
- ❑ F is useful in the investigation of anal fistula
- ❑ G cannot be used with intestinal staplers

1.52   A diabetic patient requiring abdominal surgery

☐   A   will need insulin via a sliding scale
☐   B   should be put in the middle of the list to allow the blood
            sugars to stabilise
☐   C   is prone to infection
☐   D   requires a pre-operative ECG
☐   E   should have their chlorpropamide stopped on the morning of
            surgery

**1.53   The following are suitable investigations for a 30-year-old
         woman on NSAIDs with an acute abdomen:**

☐   A   plain abdominal X-ray
☐   B   erect chest X-ray
☐   C   left lateral decubitus film
☐   D   ultrasound upper abdomen
☐   E   barium enema

1.54   A chest X-ray is indicated prior to surgery in the following:

☐   A   all over 50 years
☐   B   all over 65 years
☐   C   all recent immigrants
☐   D   all patients with malignant disease
☐   E   pre cardiac surgery

1.55   Polyglactin sutures

☐   A   are rapidly absorbed
☐   B   cause an intense tissue reaction
☐   C   are usually monofilament
☐   D   are suitable for vascular anastomosis
☐   E   slide well in tissues

1.56   Biological sutures

❑   A   may be associated with aneurysm formation
❑   B   are easy to tie
❑   C   breakdown in a predictable way
❑   D   are relatively inert
❑   E   are associated with sinus formation
❑   F   may cause anaphylaxis

1.57   Mass abdominal closure

❑   A   follows 2:1 rule; length of suture:length of wound
❑   B   follows Goodsall's law
❑   C   is most easily performed with a continuous suture
❑   D   may be carried out using absorbable sutures
❑   E   should include both anterior and posterior rectus sheath along all of its length

1.58   A full blood count is mandatory for the following patients pre-operatively:

❑   A   an 8-year-old having an appendicectomy
❑   B   a 50-year-old male smoker
❑   C   a 30-year-old woman non-smoker
❑   D   a fit and healthy 60-year-old man
❑   E   an Afro-Caribbean 18-year-old man

1.59   An ECG should be obtained on the following patients prior to surgery:

❑   A   an asymptomatic 45-year-old
❑   B   a hypertensive 40-year-old woman
❑   C   a healthy man scheduled for a femoro-popliteal bypass
❑   D   a patient with a controlled atrial fibrillation rate of 70 per minute
❑   E   a 45-year-old man for an oesophago-gastrectomy

1.60   Keloid scars

❑ A   are more common in pigmented skin
❑ B   occur within the limits of the surgical wound
❑ C   are most common on the flexure surfaces of the limbs
❑ D   may be re-excised with good results
❑ E   may respond to pressure dressing
❑ F   can be prevented by subcuticular sutures

1.61   The skin excision margin required for a

❑ A   squamous cell carcinoma is 2 cm
❑ B   basal cell carcinoma is 1 cm
❑ C   nodular melanoma is 3 cm
❑ D   macular melanoma is 1 cm

1.62   The following are true about diathermy:

❑ A   bipolar is safe on appendages
❑ B   monopolar is safe for cutting use but not coagulation on the finger
❑ C   uses frequencies up to 100 kHz
❑ D   coagulation setting uses a pulsed current
❑ E   cutting uses a square wave current

1.63   Lasers

❑ A   produce coherent light
❑ B   use photon energy
❑ C   are usually polychromatic light
❑ D   all use visible light
❑ E   may be used to treat photosensitive tumours

1.64   In the induction of anaesthesia

☐   A   ketamine is not used with concurrent cardiac disease
☐   B   ketamine provides dissociative anaesthesia
☐   C   propofol allows rapid recovery
☐   D   thiopentone causes myocardial depression
☐   E   etomidate may cause abnormal muscle movements

1.65   The following are required for the monitoring of a ventilated patient having a general anaesthetic:

☐   A   arterial blood gases
☐   B   end tidal CO_2 monitor
☐   C FiO_2 (inspired oxygen concentration)
☐   D   pulse oximetry
☐   E   airway pressure
☐   F   arterial pressure
☐   G   central venous pressure
☐   H   ECG

1.66   Local anaesthetic agents

☐   A   block the calcium channels in nerves
☐   B   predominantly affect α fibres
☐   C   are prone to tachyphylaxis
☐   D   rely on the anionic state for their effect
☐   E   block sodium channels

1.67   The maximum safe doses for

☐   A   plain bupivacaine is 2 ml/kg
☐   B   lignocaine with adrenaline is 6 mg/kg
☐   C   bupivacaine with adrenaline is 4 mg/kg
☐   D   prilocaine 0.5% in a 70 kg man is 120 ml
☐   E   plain 1% lignocaine in 70 kg man is 25 ml

1.68   Intravenous injection of local anaesthetic agents

❑   A   causes tingling of the fingers
❑   B   gives an impending sense of doom
❑   C   causes convulsions
❑   D   causes cardiac arrhythmias
❑   E   causes cerebrovascular accidents

1.69   The following are at special risk for the development of deep vein thrombosis (DVT):

❑   A   the elderly
❑   B   women on the oral contraceptive pill
❑   C   those with a previous history of thrombosis
❑   D   patients with diabetes mellitus
❑   E   those undergoing orthopaedic procedures
❑   F   fluid depleted patients
❑   G   women receiving hormone replacement therapy
❑   H   patients with malignant disease

1.70   Routine DVT prophylaxis may include

❑   A   intravenous heparinisation
❑   B   graduated compression stockings
❑   C   'flowtron boots'
❑   D   head down tilt 15° whilst operating
❑   E   ergotamine

1.71   Spinal anaesthesia

❑   A   has a rapid onset
❑   B   provides good post-operative analgesia
❑   C   may be 'topped up' in the post-operative period
❑   D   seldom causes a fall in the blood pressure
❑   E   is unlikely to cause headache

1.72   Brachial plexus block

- ❑   A   is easily performed
- ❑   B   may be complicated by a pneumothorax
- ❑   C   may cause arterial puncture
- ❑   D   may be used for post-operative pain relief
- ❑   E   may be approached via a supraclavicular route
- ❑   F   is suitable for axillary dissection
- ❑   G   is suitable for forearm surgery

1.73   The following are contraindications to epidural analgesia:

- ❑   A   severe liver disease
- ❑   B   diastematomyelia
- ❑   C   sepsis
- ❑   D   obstetric trauma
- ❑   E   neurological disease
- ❑   F   shock
- ❑   G   coagulation disorder
- ❑   H   aspirin

1.74   In premedication prior to general anaesthesia

- ❑   A   benzodiazepines provide pre-emptive analgesia
- ❑   B   benzodiazepines are good anxiolytics
- ❑   C   omnopon and scopolamine cause a distressing dry mouth
- ❑   D   omnopon and scopolamine provide good sedation
- ❑   E   omnopon and scopolamine may cause retention of urine

1.75   The following are especially at risk from sedation:

- ❑   A   children
- ❑   B   the elderly
- ❑   C   obese patients
- ❑   D   patients with an acute gastro-intestinal bleed
- ❑   E   patients with co-existent cardio-respiratory disease

1.76   Appropriate methods of biopsy include

❑   A   'Trucut' concentric needle biopsy of suspected testicular
             tumours
❑   B   cold-cup biopsy of lesions in the common bile duct
❑   C   open biopsy of suspected malignant muscle tumours
❑   D   sigmoidoscopic cold-cup biopsy suspected in Hirschsprung's
             disease

1.77   The patient should be fasted for six hours prior to

❑   A   excision of a mole on the face under local anaesthesia
❑   B   hernia repair under general anaesthesia
❑   C   hernia repair under spinal analgesia
❑   D   hernia repair under local analgesia
❑   E   colonoscopy under sedation
❑   F   femoral angiography

1.78   The following are true concerning Bier's block:

❑   A   bupivacaine should be used to provide a prolonged effect
❑   B   flumazenil should always be available
❑   C   the patient trolley used should have a tilt facility
❑   D   oxygen should be available
❑   E   cardiac monitoring is essential

**1.79   Advantages of the use of adrenaline with local anaesthetics
              include**

❑   A   potentiating the effects of the anaesthetic
❑   B   allowing a larger dose to be used
❑   C   reducing the volume of agent needed in digital blocks
❑   D   reducing bleeding
❑   E   increasing absorption of the local anaesthetic and so
             increasing the clearance

CORE MODULE 2: PERIOPERATIVE MANAGEMENT 2

2.1 **A patient on long-term high-dose prednisolone undergoing a right hemi-colectomy**

❏ A   is at increased risk of wound breakdown
❏ B   should be covered with only a single dose of intravenous hydrocortisone pre-operatively
❏ C   is at a higher risk of bleeding during the procedure
❏ D   should not have thromboprophylaxis
❏ E   has a poorer long-term prognosis than a patient not taking steroids
❏ F   requires post-operative ventilation

2.2 **In the phases of wound repair**

❏ A   coagulation cascade forms the first response
❏ B   macrophage accumulation occurs within hours
❏ C   matrix deposition is maximal after seven days
❏ D   remodelling begins after one day
❏ E   inflammatory phase rarely continues beyond ten days

2.3 **Factors delaying anastomotic healing following sigmoid colectomy include**

❏ A   tension at the anastomosis
❏ B   good blood supply
❏ C   zinc deficiency
❏ D   contamination with faecal residue
❏ E   steroids
❏ F   vitamin A deficiency

2.4   A 200 ml bolus of Haemacell

❏   A   produces a sustained (five minutes) rise of 2 cmH$_2$O in a
           dehydrated patient
❏   B   produces an initial rise and fall in CVP in a dehydrated patient
❏   C   can produce the same intravascular expansion as one litre of
           normal saline
❏   D   producing a sustained CVP rise of greater than 4 cmH$_2$O may
           indicate overfilling
❏   E   may produce anaphylactic shock

2.5   Haemacel

❏   A   remains within the intravascular space for twelve hours
❏   B   contains ten times more calcium than gelofusin
❏   C   interferes with cross-matching of blood
❏   D   should not be used as fluid challenge in cases of poor urine
           output
❏   E   is a solution of degraded starch
❏   F   is a blood product

2.6   Pulmonary aspiration

❏   A   may manifest as post-operative pneumonia
❏   B   may lead to ARDS
❏   C   complicates acute gastric dilatation
❏   D   usually occurs one week post-operatively
❏   E   may require IPPV
❏   F   can be treated with surfactant

2.7   **A 70 kg man**

❑   A   has approximately 30 litres of water distributed in the
          intracellular space
❑   B   has approximately 20 litres of water distributed in the
          interstitial space
❑   C   loses approximately 400 ml of water per day through
          respiration
❑   D   has a normal daily requirement of 60 mmol/day of potassium
❑   E   has a normal daily requirement of 50 g/day of nitrogen
          (amino acids)

2.8   **Fresh frozen plasma (FFP)**

❑   A   can only be stored for three weeks
❑   B   once thawed should be administered immediately
❑   C   should be ABO blood group compatible
❑   D   is used to reverse warfarin anticoagulation
❑   E   is used to correct hypovolaemia
❑   F   can be used to treat von Willebrand's disease

2.9   **The following are side-effects of cyclosporin:**

❑   A   skin problems
❑   B   hypotension
❑   C   gingival hypertrophy
❑   D   diabetes
❑   E   malignant change

2.10   **The immune response can be reduced by the following:**

❑   A   uraemia
❑   B   HIV infection
❑   C   jaundice
❑   D   advanced malignancy
❑   E   aspirin toxicity

2.11   With regard to organ transplantation

- [ ] A   the HLA system is carried on the short arm of chromosome 9
- [ ] B   HLA class 1 are identified by microcytotoxicity tests
- [ ] C   the one year survival for class 1 and 2 matched grafts is 90%
- [ ] D   five year rejection in complete mismatch is 35%
- [ ] E   DR and DP are class 1 antigens

2.12   Side-effects of steroids include

- [ ] A   avascular necrosis of bone
- [ ] B   pancreatitis
- [ ] C   hepatotoxicity
- [ ] D   psychosis
- [ ] E   bone marrow suppression

2.13   The following are true about wound healing:

- [ ] A   wounds may contract to up to 80%
- [ ] B   cytokines are vital to full healing
- [ ] C   vitamin D is important
- [ ] D   high wound mobility increases healing
- [ ] E   zinc accelerates healing

2.14   Signs of an anastomotic leak after anterior resection of the rectum include

- [ ] A   pyrexia
- [ ] B   increased white blood count
- [ ] C   reduced alkaline phosphatase levels
- [ ] D   increasing pain
- [ ] E   vomiting

2.15   Peripheral vein parenteral nutrition

❑   A   feeds contain solutions of similar osmolality to central venous total parenteral nutrition (TPN)
❑   B   can be given for up to ten days
❑   C   is a safer route than central venous TPN
❑   D   has improved with the availability of lipid emulsions
❑   E   should be administered via an infusion pump

2.16   Suitable dressings

❑   A   thyroidectomy
❑   B   hernia repair
❑   C   incision and drainage abscess
❑   D   varicose vein avulsions
❑   E   haemorrhoidectomy

For each of the procedures listed above, select the most appropriate dressing from the list below.

1.   pressure dressing
2.   alginate ribbon
3.   none
4.   non adherent
5.   paraffin ribbon

2.17   In haemophilia A

❑   A   epistaxis is common
❑   B   the disorder may present in the first month of life
❑   C   the bleeding time is prolonged
❑   D   cryoprecipitate from stored blood will arrest haemorrhage
❑   E   the partial thromboplastin time is normal

2.18   Early features of an incompatible blood transfusion include

- ❑   A   nausea
- ❑   B   dyspnoea
- ❑   C   jaundice
- ❑   D   myoglobinuria
- ❑   E   lumbar pain
- ❑   F   pancreatitis
- ❑   G   fever

2.19   Drains

- ❑   A   Yates
- ❑   B   Wallace/Robinson
- ❑   C   corrugated
- ❑   D   Redivac
- ❑   E   sump

For each of the drains listed above please select the best descriptive term from below.

1.   closed vacuum
2.   open
3.   closed tube
4.   irrigating
5.   tube open

2.20   Subclavian vein cannulation

- ❑   A   has a higher incidence of catheter sepsis compared with jugular vein cannulation
- ❑   B   has a lower incidence of pneumothorax compared with jugular vein cannulation
- ❑   C   may be complicated by air embolism
- ❑   D   is the preferred route for prolonged intravenous feeding
- ❑   E   is performed by insertion below the midpoint of the clavicle towards the jugular notch

2.21   Low molecular weight heparin

❑   A   neutralises activated factor V
❑   B   has a longer plasma half life compared with unfractionated
           heparin
❑   C   may be used in the treatment of DVT on an out-patient basis
❑   D   is neutralised by platelet factor 4
❑   E   must be monitored by measurement of APTT assay

2.22   Wound closure

❑   A   hernia wound
❑   B   abscess drainage incision
❑   C   abdominal wound post faeculant peritonitis
❑   D   burns to face
❑   E   circumferential burns

For each of the wounds listed above, select the most appropriate action
from below.

1.   escharotomy
2.   secondary intention
3.   primary closure
4.   excision and grafting
5.   delayed primary closure

2.23   Post-operative retention of urine

❑   A   is commoner in men
❑   B   is frequently painful
❑   C   may present with disorientation
❑   D   is common after epidural anaesthesia
❑   E   is a rare complication of haemorrhoidectomy
❑   F   may be treated with 40 mg i.v. frusemide
❑   G   may be treated with finasteride
❑   H   may be treated with bethanechol

2.24   In considering nutritional support

❑   A   parenteral nutrition has an overall lower rate of sepsis than
            enteral nutrition
❑   B   peripheral parenteral nutrition may be used for longer than
            two weeks
❑   C   enteral nutrition may be protective against multi-organ failure
❑   D   TPN is associated with zinc deficiency
❑   E   total parenteral nutrition (TPN) may be complicated by
            cholestasis

2.25   5% dextrose intravenous infusion

❑   A   is isotonic on administration
❑   B   stays within the extracellular space
❑   C   is a good mode of resuscitation in the shocked patient
❑   D   may give rise to Type II respiratory failure
❑   E   of 200 ml (bolus) will raise the CVP by 2 cm of water in a
            70 kg man
❑   F   contains 180 mmol dextrose
❑   G   contains 60 Kcal/L

2.26   The following are complications of burns:

❑   A   myoglobinuria
❑   B   hypoglycaemia
❑   C   hyponatraemia
❑   D   heterotrophic calcification
❑   E   acute appendicitis

2.27   Autologous blood

- ❑ A   transfusion prevents allergic reactions
- ❑ B   transfusion avoids all the risks of blood transfusion
- ❑ C   is contraindicated in severe cardiorespiratory disease
- ❑ D   may be donated when the patient is pyrexial
- ❑ E   may be stored for up to six months before operation

2.28   Glomerular filtration rate (GFR)

- ❑ A   declines with age
- ❑ B   may be measured with insulin clearance
- ❑ C   may be estimated by creatinine clearance
- ❑ D   is unaffected by a protein rich meal
- ❑ E   decreases during pregnancy

2.29   Metabolic acidosis occurs in

- ❑ A   vomiting
- ❑ B   hyperaldosteronism
- ❑ C   diabetes mellitus
- ❑ D   renal failure
- ❑ E   hyperparathyroidism
- ❑ F   septic shock
- ❑ G   enterocutaneous small bowel fistula

2.30   Respiratory acidosis occurs as a result of

- ❑ A   pneumonia
- ❑ B   crushing chest injury
- ❑ C   excessive mechanical ventilation
- ❑ D   pulmonary embolus
- ❑ E   head injury
- ❑ F   tracheostomy

2.31 Hyponatraemia may occur

- ❏ A with excess steroids
- ❏ B in burns
- ❏ C in fever
- ❏ D in renal failure
- ❏ E following TURP
- ❏ F with beta-adrenergic blocking agents
- ❏ G in intestinal obstruction
- ❏ H in pyloric stenosis

2.32 With regard to head injuries with a skull fracture

- ❏ A and a normal Glasgow coma scale the risk of serious intracranial injury is 1/32
- ❏ B and a reduced Glasgow coma scale the risk of serious intracranial injury is 1/2
- ❏ C the fracture can be diagnosed on one view
- ❏ D alcohol ingestion and a normal Glasgow coma scale needs CT scan
- ❏ E every patient must have a CT scan

2.33 Disseminated intravascular coagulation (DIC)

- ❏ A is always secondary to another disease process
- ❏ B may lead to ARDS
- ❏ C is associated with malignancy
- ❏ D leads to elevated levels of anti-thrombin III
- ❏ E causes decreased levels of fibrinogen degradation products

2.34   von Willebrand's disease

❑   A   is an autosomal recessive disorder
❑   B   produces a prolongation of the bleeding time
❑   C   does not affect the prothrombin time
❑   D   commonly presents with haemarthrosis
❑   E   may be treated pre-operatively with desmopressin to increase
            factor VIII and vWF levels

2.35   The following are highly suggestive of cardiac contusion following trauma:

❑   A   abnormal thallium scan
❑   B   raised creatinine kinase
❑   C   ST elevation on ECG
❑   D   tented T waves on ECG
❑   E   flail chest

2.36   Analgesia

❑   A   oral co-proxamol
❑   B   epidural catheter
❑   C   20 ml 1% local anaesthetic
❑   D   75 mg intramuscular pethidine
❑   E   patient controlled analgesia

For each of the operations below, select the most appropriate pain relief
from above.

1.   caesarean section
2.   hernia repair
3.   circumcision
4.   left hemi-colectomy
5.   pancreatitis

2.37   Blood donated for blood transfusion in the U.K. is routinely tested for

❑   A   HIV type 1
❑   B   gonorrhoea
❑   C   hepatitis C
❑   D   cytomegalovirus
❑   E   hepatitis B
❑   F   toxoplasmosis
❑   G   syphilis
❑   H   MRSA

2.38   Massive blood transfusion in the absence of immunological reaction is associated with the following complications:

❑   A   hypocalcaemia
❑   B   metabolic alkalosis
❑   C   hypothermia
❑   D   thrombocytopenia
❑   E   disseminated intravascular coagulation
❑   F   hypokalaemia

2.39   A raised MCV is seen in

❑   A   alcohol abuse
❑   B   renal failure
❑   C   thalassaemia
❑   D   iron deficiency
❑   E   paraproteinaemia

2.40   With regard to post-operative pain relief

❑   A   oral analgesia is usually satisfactory after laparotomy
❑   B   PCA should use fentanyl and an antiemetic
❑   C   bupivacaine is used because it has the fewest side-effects
❑   D   wound catheters increase infection rates
❑   E   epidural catheters using fentanyl avoid respiratory suppression

2.41   Regarding surgical complications of sickle cell disease (SCD)

❑   A   splenectomy is usually required
❑   B   there is a characteristic retinopathy
❑   C   proctitis is common
❑   D   post-operative wound infection rate is increased
❑   E   there is an acute chest syndrome

2.42   Patients with sickle cell disease worldwide

❑   A   often present with haematemesis
❑   B   have target cells in the blood
❑   C   have some normal HbA
❑   D   have a substitution of valine for glutamic acid
❑   E   have no HbF

**2.43   Prolonged irrigation with an isotonic, non-electrolytic
            solution during transurethral prostatectomy may cause**

❑   A   haemolysis
❑   B   hypoglycaemia
❑   C   hypokalaemia
❑   D   hypocalcaemia
❑   E   metabolic alkalosis

2.44   Classification of surgical wounds

❑   A   inguinal hernia repair
❑   B   perforated diverticular disease with paracolic abscess
❑   C   laparoscopic cholecystectomy
❑   D   pilonidal abscess
❑   E   thyroidectomy
❑   F   peritonitis from recent perforated duodenal ulcer
❑   G   tracheostomy

For each of the wounds listed above select the single most appropriate condition from below.

1.   clean
2.   potential contamination
3.   actual contamination
4.   dirty

3.1 In an adult male

- ❑ A blood loss 1.3 litre
- ❑ B blood loss 1.7 litre
- ❑ C blood loss 2.5 litre
- ❑ D blood loss 0.75 litre
- ❑ E blood loss 1 litre

For each of the above volumes of blood loss, select the most appropriate physiological change.

1. normal heart rate
2. unconscious
3. reduced systolic pressure
4. pale colour
5. raised diastolic pressure

3.2 The following are features of a tension pneumothorax:

- ❑ A tracheal deviation towards the affected side
- ❑ B increased chest movement on the affected side
- ❑ C increased resonance of affected side
- ❑ D cardiac arrest
- ❑ E surgical emphysema

3.3 The following are true concerning chest trauma:

- ❑ A a flail segment will give rise to Cullen's sign
- ❑ B rib fracture may be treated safely with local anaesthesia
- ❑ C rib fractures can be treated safely with an epidural catheter
- ❑ D a flail segment needs no surgical treatment
- ❑ E small pneumothoraces need no treatment

3.4 Burns covering 30% of the body surface area in an adult

- ❑ A require aggressive fluid resuscitation with crystalloids in the first 24 hours
- ❑ B may be complicated by ARDS
- ❑ C should be treated immediately with antibiotics
- ❑ D may require enteral feeding
- ❑ E are associated with a 60% mortality

3.5 The following staff should be present in the casualty department in a major incident:

- ❑ A A&E consultant
- ❑ B senior orthopaedic surgeon
- ❑ C senior administrator
- ❑ D medical houseman
- ❑ E radiologist

3.6 Nasotracheal intubation

- ❑ A can provide a definitive airway in a person with a cervical spine fracture
- ❑ B is contraindicated in the apnoeic patient
- ❑ C is a useful intubation technique in patients with base of skull fracture
- ❑ D is contraindicated in a Le Fort II fracture
- ❑ E is not used in conscious patients

3.7 **The following measurements are considered to be the upper limit of normal on lateral cervical spine films in adults:**

❏ A a distance of ≤ 5 mm from the posterior aspect of the anterior arch of the atlas to the front of the odontoid peg (the predental space)

❏ B a difference in height between the anterior and posterior aspect of a vertebral body < 4 mm

❏ C depth of the prevertebral soft tissue above the larynx ≤ 10 mm

❏ D depth of the prevertebral soft tissue space below the larynx ≤ 25 mm

❏ E depth of the spinal canal > 10 mm

3.8 **Features of a traumatic injury suggesting the possibility that a victim has sustained a major trauma include**

❏ A fall of more than 10 feet

❏ B ejection of the victim from a vehicle

❏ C extrication time > 1 hour

❏ D impact velocity > 50 mph

❏ E death of an occupant of the same vehicle

3.9 **In immediate airway management of the multiply injured patient**

❏ A nasotracheal intubation may be considered for a spontaneously breathing unconscious patient

❏ B a cricothyroidotomy is indicated after failed endotracheal intubation

❏ C the airway should be opened initially by extending the neck and performing a jaw thrust manoeuvre

❏ D a clinical base of skull fracture is a contraindication for a nasopharyngeal airway

❏ E nasal prongs can be used to deliver oxygen in the spontaneously breathing patient

3.10 Peripheral nerves

- ❏ A carry motor impulses from the spinothalamic tract
- ❏ B carry vasomotor fibres from the sympathetic chain
- ❏ C under pressure cause tingling after five minutes
- ❏ D carry sensory fibres to the posterior root ganglia
- ❏ E neurapraxia leads to permanent damage

3.11 In nerve damage

- ❏ A axonotmesis occurs after closed fractures
- ❏ B due to axonotmesis the endoneurium is disrupted
- ❏ C Wallerian degeneration may take weeks to occur
- ❏ D axons grow at 1–3 mm per day
- ❏ E neuromata may occur

3.12 With regard to neurotmesis

- ❏ A it leads to normal functional recovery
- ❏ B Wallerian degeneration occurs
- ❏ C the nerve heals with scarring
- ❏ D it may be caused by intra-neural injections
- ❏ E the endoneurium remains intact

3.13 In adult basic life support

- ❏ A for single rescuer CPR the ratio of compressions to breaths is 5:2
- ❏ B the correct compression rate is approximately 60 per minute
- ❏ C for compressions the heel of the hand should be placed over the mid sternum
- ❏ D after identifying that the victim is not breathing three rescue breaths should be given
- ❏ E visible movement of the chest indicates adequate ventilation

3.14 **The following anatomical differences in children make management of their airway more difficult than in adults:**

❑ A a more caudally placed larynx
❑ B smaller angle of the jaw
❑ C more 'U' shaped epiglottis
❑ D relatively larger tongue
❑ E larger head size compared to the body size

3.15 **During resuscitation for multisystem trauma**

❑ A supplementary oxygen should be administered by simple face mask
❑ B transfusion of unmatched type-specific blood is preferred to type O negative for life-threatening blood loss
❑ C insertion of a urinary catheter should be delayed in the presence of scrotal haematoma
❑ D the electrocardiogram should be monitored for dysrhythmias
❑ E hypovolaemia is treated with vasopressor agents

3.16 **A 20-year-old motorcyclist has collided with a tree at 70 miles per hour. He has an obvious head injury and has been transferred to your care one hour after the injury. He has been anaesthetised and ventilated. He has a blood pressure of 90/55, and a pulse of 80. Which of the following may be the cause of his hypotension?**

❑ A anaesthetic drugs
❑ B septic shock
❑ C haemorrhagic shock
❑ D neurogenic shock
❑ E extradural haematoma

3.17   Tachycardia in response to haemorrhage may be absent in the following:

❏   A   hypothermia
❏   B   infants
❏   C   patients with a pacemaker
❏   D   after administration of high flow oxygen
❏   E   patients on beta-blockers

3.18   In brachial plexus injuries

❏   A   Erb's palsy is due to a lower root lesion
❏   B   Klumpke's palsy causes clawing of the hand
❏   C   Horner's syndrome is more common with upper root lesions
❏   D   preganglionic lesions are more amenable to repair
❏   E   one must always exclude a cervical spine fracture

3.19   The following are true:

❏   A   damage to the spinal accessory nerve causes winging of the scapula
❏   B   the axillary nerve contains fibres of C6, C7
❏   C   radial nerve injuries cause wrist drop
❏   D   a positive Froment's test is associated with median nerve injury
❏   E   sciatic nerve injuries are associated with a high stepping gait

3.20   With regard to the healing of fractures

❏   A   callus formation is the first stage
❏   B   the bone edges die back for up to 15 mm
❏   C   initial bone formed is lamellar bone
❏   D   callus is involved in both deposition and resorption of bone
❏   E   remodelling can occur for many years after a fracture

3.21 Non-union of fractures is caused by

- ❑ A relative hypothermia of the fracture site
- ❑ B separation of the fracture fragments
- ❑ C interposition of tissue
- ❑ D multiple bone fragments
- ❑ E poor blood supply

3.22 Internal fixation should be used

- ❑ A where fast healing is required
- ❑ B where large forces are working in opposite directions
- ❑ C in a multiple injured patient
- ❑ D with compound fractures
- ❑ E with pathological fractures

3.23 Concerning subdural haemorrhage

- ❑ A the commonest cause is middle meningeal artery bleeds
- ❑ B it is more common in alcoholics
- ❑ C it is more common when there is an increased subdural space
- ❑ D it may be associated with minimal trauma
- ❑ E it may have no localising signs

3.24 Concerning the Glasgow Coma Scale

- ❑ A it is graded out of 14
- ❑ B abnormal flexion scores 3
- ❑ C confused verbal responses score 3
- ❑ D eye opening to pain scores 2
- ❑ E incomprehensible sounds on verbal assessment score 3

3.25   The following are true:

❑   A   a skull fracture on X-ray is diagnostic of intra-cranial injury
❑   B   air fluid levels in sinuses are diagnostic of fractures
❑   C   CT scanning is very sensitive for the diagnosis of fractures
❑   D   basal skull fractures are associated with the racoon eye sign
❑   E   petrous fractures are associated with III nerve palsies

3.26   A surgical airway

❑   A   is indicated in fracture of the larynx
❑   B   is indicated in a large extradural haematoma
❑   C   is indicated in severe oropharyngeal haemorrhage
❑   D   may be performed by a needle through the thyrohyoid membrane
❑   E   may be complicated by oesophageal perforation

3.27   After an acute 1000 ml blood loss, a 70 kg male would exhibit the following signs:

❑   A   a widened pulse pressure
❑   B   a normal blood pressure
❑   C   a respiratory rate >35 breaths per minute
❑   D   a pulse rate >100/min
❑   E   severe confusion

3.28   Concerning resuscitation fluids

❑   A   normal (physiological saline or 0.9%) contains 145 mmol/litre sodium
❑   B   Hartmann's solution contains 10 mmol/litre potassium
❑   C   Gelofusine may be infused into the same line as blood
❑   D   Haemacel is derived from gelatin
❑   E   Pentastarch has a shorter duration of action in the circulation than albumin

3.29　　**The early response to trauma (low flow or ebb phase) includes**

❑　A　increase in metabolic rate
❑　B　increase in body temperature
❑　C　increase in catecholamine levels
❑　D　decreased lactate levels
❑　E　increased glucose levels

3.30　　**A 30-year-old female has been stabbed in the left chest. She is short of breath, has a pulse of 120 and a systolic blood pressure of 80 mmHg. Which of the following statements are true?**

❑　A　the presence of distended neck veins with good bilateral air entry would warrant an immediate pericardiocentesis
❑　B　hyper-resonance to percussion over the left chest, with tracheal deviation to the right would warrant immediate needle thoracocentesis to the left chest
❑　C　she requires immediate thoracotomy
❑　D　a chest X-ray is required before any invasive procedure
❑　E　a central venous pressure measurement will distinguish between a tension pneumothorax and a cardiac tamponade

3.31　　**In subarachnoid haemorrhage**

❑　A　the most common cause is an aneurysm
❑　B　diagnosis is made on non-contrast CT in the first 48 hours
❑　C　calcium channel blockers should be given to counteract vasospasm
❑　D　early surgery should be considered for patients in a poor neurological condition
❑　E　5% of patients with an aneurysmal origin will have multiple aneurysms

3.32   The effects of haemorrhage due to trauma

❏   A   are very poorly tolerated by the older patient
❏   B   may be masked by beta-blockers
❏   C   are unaffected by hypothermia
❏   D   are determined by pre-existing cardiovascular status of the patient
❏   E   may be monitored by CVP

3.33   The following are true concerning skull fractures:

❏   A   patients with simple skull fractures do not need antibiotics
❏   B   meningitis is associated with NG and ET intubation and CSF leaks
❏   C   meningitis in fractures is usually the result of infection from faecal flora
❏   D   meningitis is associated with normal commensal CSF flora
❏   E   patients with large CSF leaks should be nursed in the sitting position

3.34   Intraosseous infusion

❏   A   is routinely indicated in paediatric trauma
❏   B   can be used in children up to the age of 12 years
❏   C   is performed by the Seldinger technique
❏   D   is carried out by puncture on the surface of the tibia
❏   E   should be discontinued when other venous access has been obtained

3.35   Indications for a skull X-ray after head injury include

❏   A   rhinorrhoea
❏   B   alcohol intoxication
❏   C   epileptics in a post ictal state
❏   D   large scalp contusions and lacerations
❏   E   patients who have had a previous craniotomy

3.36 Acute spinal cord transection at the level of C6

- ❑ A is associated with apnoea
- ❑ B is associated with progressive hypoxia
- ❑ C results in hypertension
- ❑ D results in tachycardia
- ❑ E results in arreflexia

3.37 Peripheral venous cutdown

- ❑ A may be to the long saphenous vein 2 cm posterior and superior to the medial malleolus
- ❑ B may be to the subclavian vein
- ❑ C may be to the medial basilic vein
- ❑ D may be complicated by cellulitis
- ❑ E does not allow adequate volume replacement

3.38 Tension pneumothorax

- ❑ A is most commonly seen in ventilated patients
- ❑ B causes a shift of the trachea towards the affected side
- ❑ C produces a positive Kussmaul's sign
- ❑ D is diagnosed by chest X-ray
- ❑ E produces similar features to cardiac tamponade

3.39 The following are true of brain death:

- ❑ A it may be caused by increased intra-cranial pressure
- ❑ B it is not related to brain stem events
- ❑ C it is diagnosed by apnoea despite reduced pCO_2
- ❑ D diagnosis may be made irrespective of concurrent medication
- ❑ E diagnosis must be made by two independent consultants

3.40   With respect to spinal injury the following are true:

- ❏ A   quadriplegia and paraplegia are equally common
- ❏ B   thoraco-lumbar injury is the most common
- ❏ C   urinary incontinence is common on presentation and of little significance
- ❏ D   it may mask other injuries
- ❏ E   it takes priority in triage

3.41   The following are true of chest trauma:

- ❏ A   massive haemothorax may be difficult to diagnose on chest X-ray
- ❏ B   the main effect of a tension pneumothorax is respiratory
- ❏ C   massive haemothorax needs immediate surgical exploration
- ❏ D   tension pneumothorax should be diagnosed on a chest X-ray
- ❏ E   tension pneumothorax may present with surgical emphysema

3.42   Major accident plan for the oncall surgeon includes

- ❏ A   reporting to the manager of the operating theatres
- ❏ B   on arrival at disaster, go to the ambulance control vehicle
- ❏ C   changing into clothing, including orange tabard
- ❏ D   the emergency box should contain an amputation set
- ❏ E   the emergency box should contain a tracheostomy set and a Heimlich valve

3.43   To calculate the Revised Trauma Score which of the following parameters are required?

- ❏ A   pulse pressure
- ❏ B   Glasgow Coma Score
- ❏ C   pulse rate
- ❏ D   systolic blood pressure
- ❏ E   respiratory rate

3.44   Regarding the Injury Severity Score

- ❏   A   the Injury Severity Score is the sum of the squares of the three highest abbreviated injury scale scores in the three most severely affected regions of the body
- ❏   B   an Abbreviated Injury Scale score of 6 indicates an injury which is virtually unsurvivable
- ❏   C   the body surface is one of the designated regions used in the Injury Severity Score
- ❏   D   an Injury Severity Score of > 10 denotes a major trauma
- ❏   E   the maximum Injury Severity Score is 70

3.45   Split thickness skin grafts

- ❏   A   survive well when placed over blood clots
- ❏   B   require the application of direct pressure to 'take'
- ❏   C   are best suited to well vascularised clean wounds
- ❏   D   commonly fail when applied to the back
- ❏   E   should be taken from a donor area that matches in colour and texture

3.46   The following are true concerning maxillofacial trauma:

- ❏   A   a chest X-ray is mandatory
- ❏   B   if the mouth is involved then the patient will need intubation
- ❏   C   tracheostomy can be performed in the casualty department if an airway cannot be established
- ❏   D   Le Fort I fractures involve the inferior orbital rim
- ❏   E   Le Fort II fractures cause malocclusion

3.47   The following are true:

❑   A   the skull is thickest in the antero-inferior region
❑   B   the dura mater is most exterior
❑   C   the arachnoid mater allows passage of important arteries
❑   D   the pia mater forms a tough sheath
❑   E   CSF is found exterior to the dura mater

3.48   Aortic rupture may be suggested by

❑   A   a widened mediastinum
❑   B   a prominent aortic knuckle
❑   C   radiofemoral delay
❑   D   depression of the right main-stem bronchus
❑   E   tracheal deviation to the right
❑   F   deviation of a nasogastric tube in the oesophagus to the right

3.49   Traumatic diaphragmatic hernia should be suspected if there

❑   A   is an air fluid level in the chest
❑   B   is a pneumomediastinum
❑   C   are signs of intestinal obstruction after injury
❑   D   is fracture in the first three ribs
❑   E   is unclear outline of the diaphragm

3.50   Diagnostic peritoneal lavage

❑   A   is 85% sensitive for intraperitoneal bleeding
❑   B   is relatively contraindicated in morbid obesity
❑   C   should not be performed if there is peritonitis
❑   D   can exclude a retroperitoneal injury
❑   E   can provide information about specific organ injury

3.51 Acute extradural haematoma

- ❏ A is a common sequelae of head injury
- ❏ B may occur from a tear in the dural sinus
- ❏ C produces a lucid interval
- ❏ D produces a contralateral dilated fixed pupil
- ❏ E has a mortality of 50% in the non-comatose patient
- ❏ F is usually due to middle meningeal artery injury
- ❏ G is rare in the absence of a skull fracture

3.52 With regard to healing of fractures of tubular bones

- ❏ A the process of fracture healing occurs in five stages, starting with the fracture haematoma
- ❏ B cell proliferation at the fracture site occurs late in the healing of fractures
- ❏ C the woven bone is transformed to lamellar bone by the osteoblasts
- ❏ D the callus at the fracture site is less profuse in children
- ❏ E bone remodelling in children after a fracture is so perfect that eventually the site of the fracture becomes indistinguishable in radiographs

3.53 The following are true concerning complications of fractures:

- ❏ A the incidence of myositis ossificans is increased by open surgery
- ❏ B late rupture of abductor pollicis longus is seen in Colles' fracture
- ❏ C fractures of the shaft of the humerus are associated with wrist drop
- ❏ D compartment syndrome presents early with paraesthesia
- ❏ E damage to the lateral popliteal nerve is a recognised complication of tibial plateau fracture

3.54   Early findings in compartment syndrome include

- ❏   A   paraesthesia
- ❏   B   absent distal pulses
- ❏   C   pink skin
- ❏   D   pain on passively stretching the affected muscles
- ❏   E   'pressure feeling' in limbs

3.55   Compartment syndrome

- ❏   A   is more common in open than closed fractures
- ❏   B   is rare in the upper limb
- ❏   C   can be managed conservatively with intravenous heparin
- ❏   D   can be excluded in the presence of palpable pulses
- ❏   E   leads to Volkmann's ischaemic contracture

3.56   A cervical cord injury should be suspected in an unconscious patient if there is

- ❏   A   grimacing to pain above the clavicle
- ❏   B   increased upper body tone
- ❏   C   priapism
- ❏   D   hypotension with bradycardia
- ❏   E   ability to extend the elbow

3.57   Maxillofacial trauma

- ❏   A   is commonly associated with cervical spine injury
- ❏   B   is most often due to RTA in the UK
- ❏   C   to the maxilla is associated with hooding of the eye
- ❏   D   may be associated with superior orbital fissure syndrome
- ❏   E   causing an isolated Le Fort III may be associated with neurotmesis of the infraorbital nerve

3.58   Following trauma, there is

☐ A   increased muscle glycogen breakdown
☐ B   increased insulin secretion
☐ C   an elevation of blood glucose
☐ D   reduced excretion of excess water in the first 48 hours
☐ E   sodium conservation in the first 48 hours

3.59   The following are true concerning cerebro-spinal fluid:

☐ A   CSF is manufactured in cavities of the brain
☐ B   it flows between the ventricles via the aqueduct of Sylvius
☐ C   the third ventricle lies in the midbrain
☐ D   CSF is produced at a rate of 2 ml/hr
☐ E   CSF is produced by the arachnoid villi

3.60   Cerebral blood flow

☐ A   fluctuates widely from lying to standing
☐ B   is related to intra-cranial pressure
☐ C   auto-regulates directly to arterial pCO_2
☐ D   auto-regulates directly to arterial pO_2
☐ E   is increased in the normal subject by the administration of Mannitol

3.61   Concerning extra-dural haemorrhage

☐ A   the trauma is to the dural venous system
☐ B   it may have a delayed presentation
☐ C   there is always a lucent period
☐ D   the main effect is caused through an increase in intracranial pressure
☐ E   in the majority the pupil dilates on the opposite side

CORE MODULE 4: INTENSIVE CARE

4.1   With regard to bronchiectasis

❑   A   it usually occurs in adulthood
❑   B   airway obstruction plays little role
❑   C   it usually follows measles or whooping cough
❑   D   it is associated with Kartagener's syndrome
❑   E   it may present with life-threatening haemoptysis

4.2   Intermittent Positive Pressure Ventilation (IPPV)

❑   A   enlarges the physiological dead space
❑   B   increases the functional residual capacity
❑   C   increases cardiac output
❑   D   causes an increase in lung compliance
❑   E   reduces right atrial pressure
❑   F   increases ADH secretion

4.3   Functional Residual Capacity (FRC)

❑   A   is increased in the elderly
❑   B   is measured by a helium dilution technique
❑   C   represents approximately 60% of vital capacity
❑   D   falls following abdominal surgery
❑   E   is the sum of the residual volume and expiratory reserve
          volume
❑   F   is reduced in asthma
❑   G   is increased in fibrosing alveolitis

4.4 **The oxygen-haemoglobin dissociation curve is shifted to the right by**

- [ ] A increased temperature
- [ ] B asthma
- [ ] C metabolic alkalosis
- [ ] D increased 2,3-diphosphoglyceric acid (2,3-DPG)
- [ ] E elevation of pCO_2
- [ ] F carbon monoxide poisoning

4.5 **Pulmonary embolism**

- [ ] A usually results in arterial hypercapnia
- [ ] B usually produces S1 Q3 T3 changes on ECG
- [ ] C may be diagnosed by spiral CT
- [ ] D is treated by low molecular weight heparins
- [ ] E is diagnosed by a matched ventilation perfusion defect
- [ ] F usually results in arterial hypoxia

4.6 **The following are found in the superior mediastinum:**

- [ ] A the azygous vein
- [ ] B the thymus
- [ ] C the pericardium
- [ ] D the right main bronchus
- [ ] E the left recurrent laryngeal nerve

4.7 **The following are true concerning lung sepsis:**

- [ ] A abscesses may be a result of concurrent lung malignancy
- [ ] B abscesses are unusual after aspiration
- [ ] C antibiotics are the treatment of choice in empyema
- [ ] D in empyema open drainage usually leads to problems with pneumothorax
- [ ] E antibiotics help resolution of lung abscesses

4.8   **When correctly inserting an intercostal drain the following structures are penetrated:**

- ❑ A   pectoralis major
- ❑ B   serratus anterior
- ❑ C   visceral pleura
- ❑ D   parietal pleura
- ❑ E   internal intercostal muscle
- ❑ F   transversus abdominis

4.9   **The right ventricle**

- ❑ A   is most likely to be injured in a stabbing
- ❑ B   is the most anterior heart chamber
- ❑ C   is best visualised by trans-oesophageal echo
- ❑ D   is supplied by the right coronary artery
- ❑ E   receives no blood from the lungs

4.10   **The following are complications of a dissection of the ascending aorta:**

- ❑ A   mitral valve rupture
- ❑ B   aortic regurgitation
- ❑ C   cardiac tamponade
- ❑ D   acute myocardial infarction
- ❑ E   pulmonary embolus
- ❑ F   haemothorax

4.11   **The following are branches of the left coronary artery:**

- ❑ A   right marginal artery
- ❑ B   sinu atrial artery
- ❑ C   circumflex artery
- ❑ D   anterior interventricular artery
- ❑ E   obtuse marginal artery

4.12   Atrial fibrillation may cause

❑   A   mitral stenosis
❑   B   stroke
❑   C   mesenteric infarction
❑   D   gangrene of the toes
❑   E   dyspnoea
❑   F   pulmonary embolism

4.13   Auscultation of the heart

❑   A   left anterior axillary line second intercostal space
❑   B   apex
❑   C   5th intercostal space mid clavicular line
❑   D   left sternal edge 2nd intercostal space
❑   E   right sternal edge 5th intercostal space

For each of the anatomical locations in the list above pick the single most appropriate valve from the list below.

1.   mitral valve
2.   aortic valve
3.   tricuspid valve
4.   pulmonary valve
5.   none

4.14   During a central line insertion using the right subclavian route the tip may lie in the

❑   A   superior vena cava
❑   B   inferior vena cava
❑   C   left subclavian artery
❑   D   left brachiocephalic vein
❑   E   right internal jugular vein

4.15   The following actions may have a positive inotropic effect on the heart:

❏ A   dopamine at 2 µg/kg/min
❏ B   dopamine at 10 µg/kg/min
❏ C   intravenous calcium
❏ D   intravenous frusemide
❏ E   digoxin

4.16   In the following types of shock the initial management is fluid replacement:

❏ A   cardiogenic
❏ B   hypovolaemic
❏ C   anaphylactic
❏ D   septic
❏ E   obstructive

4.17   Complications of the insertion of a central venous catheter include

❏ A   pneumothorax
❏ B   haemothorax
❏ C   embolus
❏ D   infection
❏ E   stroke
❏ F   cardiac tamponade

4.18   The following are true of the jugular venous pressure (JVP):

❏ A   it is always reduced in shock
❏ B   it is raised in cardiac tamponade
❏ C   it shows diagnostic a and v waves in atrial fibrillation
❏ D   it is measured with the patient flat from the mid axillary point
❏ E   it is reduced during CPAP ventilation

4.19   The following can be directly measured with a pulmonary artery flotation catheter:

❑   A   cardiac output
❑   B   stroke volume
❑   C   left atrial pressure
❑   D   systemic vascular resistance
❑   E   central venous pressure
❑   F   right artrial pressure
❑   G   cardiac oxygen consumption

4.20   The following are true of the coronary circulation:

❑   A   maximal during systole
❑   B   coronary arteries are end arteries
❑   C   autoregulates
❑   D   is 5 l/min
❑   E   reverses during diastole

4.21   The following cause an increase in the heart rate:

❑   A   complete cardiac denervation
❑   B   intravenous adenosine
❑   C   intravenous adrenaline
❑   D   salbutamol
❑   E   metronidazole

4.22   The following statements are true:

❑   A   adequate BP equates to tissue perfusion
❑   B   systemic vascular resistance = CVP x cardiac output
❑   C   BP = heart rate x cardiac output
❑   D   cardiac output = heart rate x stroke volume
❑   E   systemic vascular resistance = BP/cardiac output

4.23   The following are true for the infective organisms

❑   A   *Klebsiella* are Gram-negative
❑   B   *Staphylococci* are Gram-positive
❑   C   *Proteus* are Gram-positive
❑   D   *Clostridia* are Gram-negative
❑   E   *Streptococci* are Gram-negative
❑   F   *Bacteroides* are Gram-negative
❑   G   *Neisseria* are Gram-positive

4.24   Infections on the ITU may be predisposed by the following

❑   A   malignant disease
❑   B   abdominal surgery
❑   C   high FiO_2
❑   D   antibiotics
❑   E   hand washing

4.25   Appropriate antibiotic treatment

❑   A   *Staphylococcus aureus*
❑   B   *Bacteroides*
❑   C   *Haemophilus influenzae*
❑   D   Enterococci
❑   E   *Klebsiella pneumoniae*

For each of the above infections select the most appropriate antibiotic from the list below.

1.   erythromycin
2.   metronidazole
3.   flucloxacillin
4.   vancomycin
5.   amoxycillin
6.   clarithromycin
7.   teicoplanin

4.26   The following drugs are safe to use in normal doses in renal failure:

❑ A   gentamicin
❑ B   digoxin
❑ C   adenosine
❑ D   pethidine
❑ E   lactulose

4.27   The following are true for a patient with a diagnosis of sepsis:

❑ A $pCO_2 < 4.2$ kPa
❑ B   HR < 50 bpm
❑ C   WCC > 12 X 10^9/l
❑ D   WCC < 4.0 X 10^9/l
❑ E $pO_2 < 10$ kPa

4.28   In septic shock

❑ A   specific organisms give characteristic host responses
❑ B   the central venous pressure is increased
❑ C   mean arterial pressure may be normal
❑ D   the systemic vascular resistance is increased
❑ E   the cardiac output increases even though the patient may be hypotensive

4.29   The following are causes of ARDS (adult respiratory distress syndrome):

❑ A   sepsis
❑ B   fat embolism
❑ C   acute pancreatitis
❑ D   acute renal failure
❑ E   burns

4.30   In ARDS (adult respiratory distress syndrome)

☐ A lung compliance is increased
☐ B left atrial pressure is increased
☐ C the patient is tachypnoeic
☐ D there is thickening of the alveolar capillary membranes
☐ E there is a V/Q mismatch

4.31   Duration of ECG components

☐ A PR interval
☐ B QRS duration
☐ C P wave
☐ D QT interval
☐ E cardiac cycle

For each of the components in the cardiac cycle above please select the single most appropriate answer from the list below.

1.   0.12 s
2.   < 0.3 s
3.   < 0.1 s
4.   1.2 s
5.   < 0.2 s

4.32   Cardiac pressures (mmHg) expressed as systolic/diastolic

❑   A   left ventricle
❑   B   right ventricle
❑   C   left atrium
❑   D   right atrium
❑   E   pulmonary artery
❑   F   aorta

For each of the sites in the heart above please select the single most appropriate pressure reading from the list below.

1.   20/0
2.   120/80
3.   5/10
4.   0/4
5.   20/6
6.   120/0

4.33   The following are complications of acute tubular necrosis:

❑   A   atrial fibrillation
❑   B   hypokalaemia
❑   C   uraemia
❑   D   disseminated intravascular coagulopathy
❑   E   metabolic alkalosis

4.34   A 21-year-old found on the floor after a drug overdose is anuric, potential causes include

❑   A   hypotension
❑   B   acute tubular necrosis
❑   C   rhabdomyolysis
❑   D   renal calculi
❑   E   sickle cell disease

4.35   The following are true of a patient in established renal failure on the ICU:

❑   A   fluid input should be limited to 2 l/day
❑   B   a Brescia-Cimino fistula will be required
❑   C   mannitol infusion is needed
❑   D   peritoneal dialysis is needed
❑   E   a Schribner shunt is required
❑   F   haemodiafiltration is needed
❑   G   a shunt will need to be formed

4.36   In the inflammatory response

❑   A   cytokines are polysaccharides
❑   B   cytokines are released by endothelial cells
❑   C   cytokines include TNF
❑   D   polymorpho-macrophages cause direct cell damage
❑   E   cell damage may involve oxygen dependent mechanisms

4.37   Anti-inflammatory agents that have established benefit in the treatment of multi-organ dysfunction include

❑   A   TNF antibodies
❑   B   steroids
❑   C   naloxone
❑   D   NSAID
❑   E   sulfametopyrazine

4.38   A patient two days post-colectomy is found to be oliguric, you should

❑   A   administer frusemide
❑   B   administer a fluid challenge
❑   C   assess for abdominal deterioration
❑   D   check urine for casts and tubular cells
❑   E   flush urinary catheter

4.39   The following may be indicated for respiratory compromise:

❏   A   oxygen
❏   B   heparin
❏   C   methohexitone
❏   D   propranolol
❏   E   morphine

4.40   Tracheostomy

❏   A   may be carried out in an emergency under sedation
❏   B   is uncomplicated by thyroid disease
❏   C   may be needed for bronchial toilet
❏   D   is straightforward in people with a short neck
❏   E   will increase dead space
❏   F   increases the ventilation-perfusion mismatch

4.41   The following are indications for ventilation:

❏   A   inability to control the airway
❏   B $pCO_2 > 5$ kPa
❏   C   respiratory rate > 35 bpm
❏   D   poor bronchial toilet
❏   E $PaO_2 < 10$ kPa

4.42   Pulse oximetry may be misleading in

❏   A   the use of cosmetics
❏   B   shock
❏   C   acute type 1 respiratory failure
❏   D   carbon monoxide poisoning
❏   E   patients on intravenous respiratory stimulants
❏   F   anaemia

4.43   A chest X-ray must be obtained on an ICU

- ❑ A   after ET tube insertion
- ❑ B   after NG tube insertion
- ❑ C   after insertion of a central line
- ❑ D   after the insertion of a chest drain
- ❑ E   in the immediate assessment of acute severe respiratory compromise

4.44   100% oxygen treatment may be administered by

- ❑ A   CPAP
- ❑ B   normal face mask
- ❑ C   PEEP
- ❑ D   resuscitation bag with reservoir
- ❑ E   nasal speculae

4.45   Fat embolus

- ❑ A   occurs mostly after compound long bone fractures
- ❑ B   may occur following burns
- ❑ C   initially presents with confusion and dyspnoea
- ❑ D   may lead to ARDS
- ❑ E   produces characteristic petechiae around the fracture site

4.46   Paralysis of the left hemi-diaphragm

- ❑ A   is caused by section of the cord below C6
- ❑ B   is caused by section of the left phrenic nerve alone
- ❑ C   causes diaphragmatic flattening during inspiration
- ❑ D   rises on inspiration
- ❑ E   increases intrathoracic pressure on the left
- ❑ F   may occur with carcinoma of the bronchus

4.47 **In an antero-lateral thoracotomy the following muscles will be cut:**

❏ A teres minor
❏ B pectoralis minor
❏ C serratus anterior
❏ D latissimus dorsi
❏ E subscapularis

4.48 **Inspiration involves**

❏ A descent of the hemi-diaphragms
❏ B reduction of vertical dimension of the chest
❏ C upward/forward movement of the first rib
❏ D contraction of the intercostal muscles
❏ E long thoracic nerve of Bell (n. to serratus anterior)

4.49 **Anterior relations of the intra-thoracic trachea include**

❏ A arch of the aorta
❏ B thymus
❏ C right lung pleura
❏ D azygous vein
❏ E sternothyroid muscles

4.50 **Contents of the left hilum of the lung include**

❏ A pulmonary artery
❏ B main bronchus
❏ C azygous vein
❏ D left middle pulmonary vein
❏ E pulmonary ligament

4.51   Pancoast's tumour may commonly be associated with

❏   A   metastatic colonic spread
❏   B   phrenic nerve involvement
❏   C   Horner's syndrome
❏   D   T1 involvement
❏   E   basal atelectasis

4.52   Respiration involves

❏   A   negative intra-thoracic pressure
❏   B   stimulatory effect of baroreceptors
❏   C   cortical control
❏   D   cavernous sinus receptors
❏   E   C fibre receptors

4.53   Metabolic and acid-base balance

❏   A   the greatest stimulus to breathing
❏   B   pulmonary embolism
❏   C   type I respiratory failure
❏   D   tented T waves
❏   E   aspirin overdose

For the list above please select the single most appropriate metabolic disturbance from the list below.

1.   hyperkalaemia
2.   hypoxia
3.   acidosis
4.   hypercarbia
5.   hypocarbia

4.54 **The following are causes of ventilation/perfusion mismatch:**

❑ A atelectasis
❑ B pulmonary oedema
❑ C pleural effusion
❑ D pulmonary embolism
❑ E right upper/middle lobectomy
❑ F lymphangitis carcinomatosa

4.55 **In a restrictive lung disorder**

❑ A alveolar membranes are thickened
❑ B compliance is reduced
❑ C transfer factor is low
❑ D PaO_2 may be increased
❑ E lung volumes are normal

4.56 **In an obstructive lung disorder**

❑ A the main problem is inspiratory
❑ B transfer factor is reduced
❑ C total lung capacity is increased
❑ D there may be bronchial dilators
❑ E lungs are more compliant

4.57 **Following anterior resection there is**

❑ A an increased loss of sodium
❑ B a decreased loss of potassium
❑ C an increased secretion of ADH
❑ D an increased urea production
❑ E an increased urine osmolality
❑ F an increased glomerular filtration rate

4.58   Antidiuretic hormone

☐ A   is secreted by the anterior pituitary
☐ B   secretion is controlled by osmoreceptors in the hypothalamus
☐ C   decreases glomerular filtration rate
☐ D   increases the permeability of the collecting ducts of the kidney to water
☐ E   reduces sodium absorption in the loop of Henlé

4.59   Cardiac output in health

☐ A   increases with stroke volume
☐ B   is increased by intravenous calcium
☐ C   increases with increase in central venous pressure
☐ D   increases with rise in systemic arterial pressure
☐ E   may be measured using the Fick principle
☐ F   is decreased in septic shock

4.60   Hypertension in the post-operative period is commonly due to

☐ A   urinary retention
☐ B   surgical incision pain
☐ C   isofluorane
☐ D   epidural analgesia
☐ E   acute tubular necrosis
☐ F   sepsis

4.61   Heat loss during laparotomy may be minimised by

☐ A   humidification of inspired gases
☐ B   lavage with warm saline
☐ C   maintaining the environmental temperature at 20°C
☐ D   use of a water blanket set at 35°C
☐ E   use of a heat reflecting blanket

4.62   Hypokalaemia

❑   A   produces peaked T waves on ECG
❑   B   causes the heart to arrest in diastole
❑   C   is seen in metabolic acidosis
❑   D   may occur following extensive muscle trauma
❑   E   may be seen in pancreatic fistulae
❑   F   may be seen in pyloric stenosis

4.63   An arterial plasma bicarbonate level of 15 mmol/l is consistent with

❑   A   respiratory acidosis
❑   B   compensatory respiratory acidosis
❑   C   metabolic acidosis
❑   D   compensatory metabolic acidosis
❑   E   compensatory metabolic alkalosis

4.64   Following major haemorrhage due to trauma

❑   A   hyperventilation occurs
❑   B   ADH is secreted in increased amounts
❑   C   tidal volume increases
❑   D   the oxygen-haemoglobin dissociation curve shifts to the right
❑   E   an initial hyperglycaemia occurs

4.65   The following are complications of sepsis:

❑   A   hypoglycaemia
❑   B   negative nitrogen balance
❑   C   increased levels of fibrinogen degradation products
❑   D   jaundice
❑   E   gangrene

4.66   Prokinetic drugs used on ICU include

- ❑   A   cisapride
- ❑   B   erythromycin
- ❑   C   sucralfate
- ❑   D   lansoprazole
- ❑   E   octreotide
- ❑   F   mastrazole

4.67   Lung compliance

- ❑   A   is the total volume of the lungs
- ❑   B   is normally below 30 ml/cm H_2O
- ❑   C   is normally 70 ml/cm H_2O
- ❑   D   may be reduced due to abdominal pathology
- ❑   E   is calculated end tidal volume/ end inspiratory pressure

4.68   Gas transfer is routinely calculated using

- ❑   A   nitrogen
- ❑   B   carbon dioxide
- ❑   C   carbon monoxide
- ❑   D   helium
- ❑   E   oxygen
- ❑   F   corrections for lung volume

4.69   Blood gases

- ❑   A   are routinely taken from the brachial artery
- ❑   B   do not vary with temperature
- ❑   C   are affected by antibiotic administration
- ❑   D   calculate the blood bicarbonate level
- ❑   E   can tell oxygen content
- ❑   F   are affected by heparin

4.70   Complications of arterial lines include

❑ A   arteriovenous fistulae
❑ B   anaemia
❑ C   aneurysm
❑ D   gangrene
❑ E   heart block

4.71   The following are true:

❑ A $PaCO_2$ is increased in type 1 respiratory failure
❑ B PaO_2 is reduced in type 2 respiratory failure
❑ C   acute left ventricular failure causes reduced $PaCO_2$
❑ D   oxygen saturation is always a good guide to tissue oxygenation
❑ E   acidosis may occur with a high HCO_3^-

4.72   Flow volume curves

Match the following diagnoses to each of the curves shown below.

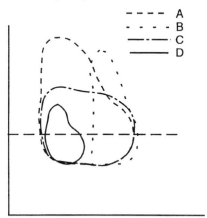

- - - - A
· - · - · B
—·—·— C
———— D

1.   upper airway obstruction
2.   normal
3.   obstructive disorder
4.   restrictive disorder

4.73   Swan-Ganz catheters

❏   A   may be used to measure cardiac output
❏   B   can measure systemic vascular resistance directly
❏   C   are only inserted via the internal jugular vein
❏   D   measure left atrial pressure
❏   E   may be complicated by pulmonary infarction

CORE MODULE 5: NEOPLASIA, TECHNIQUES AND OUTCOME OF SURGERY

5.1 The following tumours respond poorly to chemotherapy:

- ❑ A thyroid cancer
- ❑ B choriocarcinoma
- ❑ C breast cancer
- ❑ D melanoma
- ❑ E acute lymphoblastic leukaemia

5.2 In faecal occult blood tests for the diagnosis of colorectal tumours

- ❑ A the haemoccult test is dependent on the urease reaction
- ❑ B ingestion of vegetables with high peroxidase activity may cause a false-positive result
- ❑ C over 50% of asymptomatic tumours may be missed
- ❑ D they may be of use in screening family members of those with Lynch syndrome
- ❑ E they cannot identify benign adenomas

5.3 Malignant melanoma

- ❑ A should be excised with a 5 cm margin when Breslow thickness > 3 cm
- ❑ B has a better prognosis on the limb than on the trunk
- ❑ C responds well to adjuvant chemotherapy
- ❑ D may be treated with targeted gene therapy
- ❑ E rarely metastasises to lymph nodes
- ❑ F is increasing in incidence

5.4 Audit

- ❑ A is a useful research tool available to some surgeons
- ❑ B is funded largely by research funding
- ❑ C should be considered as a cycle
- ❑ D guidelines are best devised by external experts
- ❑ E process per se improves clinical practice

5.5 Audit

- ❏ A is primarily involved with outcome analysis
- ❏ B should be led by the audit department
- ❏ C is the process of peer review
- ❏ D only concerns doctors
- ❏ E process refers to what is done to the patient

5.6 In the United Kingdom breast screening programme

- ❏ A women have a single view mammogram at the first screen
- ❏ B physical examination is not carried out at the first screen
- ❏ C screens are presently repeated every two years
- ❏ D women over 65 years are no longer eligible for screening mammography
- ❏ E ductal carcinoma in situ (DCIS) is detected in 30% cases

5.7 Fine Needle Aspiration Cytology (FNAC) in the investigation of breast carcinoma

- ❏ A has a sensitivity of 95%
- ❏ B has a positive predictive value of 99.8%
- ❏ C is taken using a 14G needle
- ❏ D may be useful for assessing hormone receptor status
- ❏ E when classified as C0 signifies benign disease
- ❏ F requires local anaesthesia

5.8 Mastalgia

- ❏ A is usually cyclical
- ❏ B is most common in the third and fourth decades
- ❏ C usually presents with a discrete thickening of the breast
- ❏ D may be treated with tamoxifen
- ❏ E is usually relieved immediately when treated with evening primrose oil
- ❏ F can be treated by danazole

5.9   In the consent to treatment for minors

❏   A   the minimum legal age of consent for surgical treatment is
16 years
❏   B   a competent child aged 17 can always veto treatment which
his parents have authorised
❏   C   for patients aged 16 or 17 it is necessary to discuss the
decision with the parents
❏   D   the surgeon may undertake urgent treatment of the
unconscious child without consent

**5.10   When a patient presents acutely unconscious because of
injury**

❏   A   the surgeon may undertake life-saving treatment without
consent
❏   B   a note should be made in the clinical records to explain the
absence of formal consent
❏   C   the surgeon should confine himself to providing only
necessary treatment
❏   D   elective ventilation to preserve the organs for donation is
acceptable practice

5.11   Informed consent

❏   A   should be obtained before any sedation is given
❏   B   is the responsibility of the house officer
❏   C   may be implied
❏   D   is not valid when not written
❏   E   should be repeated if the patient's condition changes prior to
admission

5.12   Cutaneous malignant melanoma

❑ A   has a rising incidence
❑ B   has no sex predilection
❑ C   is more common on the back and face in women
❑ D   has no familial component
❑ E   is more common in higher socioeconomic groups

5.13   Radiotherapy

❑ A   is rarely used for palliation of symptoms
❑ B   given post-operatively reduces local recurrence for breast carcinoma
❑ C   given pre-operatively for rectal carcinoma reduces local recurrence in rectal cancer
❑ D   is most effective when given in a single large dose
❑ E   is less effective for slow growing tumours
❑ F   commonly causes hair loss

5.14   In the treatment of pain in the terminally ill

❑ A   diamorphine is avoided because it is addictive
❑ B   non-steroidal anti-inflammatory drugs are avoided because of the risk of gastric ulceration and haemorrhage
❑ C   the use of continuous infusion delivery systems can provide sustained pain control
❑ D   intravenous opiates are contraindicated in children
❑ E   antidepressants can be used for neurogenic pain

5.15   Alpha-fetoprotein (AFP) levels are useful in monitoring treatment of

❑   A   seminoma
❑   B   teratoma
❑   C   hepatoma
❑   D   pancreatic carcinoma
❑   E   yolk sac tumour

5.16   Serum carcinoembryonic antigen (CEA)

❑   A   is useful as it detects recurrence of colorectal cancer
❑   B   is a glycoprotein
❑   C   is raised in 90% of cases of colorectal cancer
❑   D   has a mean half-life of 100 days
❑   E   is elevated in smokers

5.17   Basal cell carcinoma of the skin

❑   A   is more common in men
❑   B   is familial
❑   C   can be treated by cryotherapy
❑   D   is classically a flat erythematous lesion with pale atrophic areas
❑   E   is usually treated with a 1 cm excision margin
❑   F   on the nose may be treated with radiotherapy
❑   G   usually metastasises to the regional lymph nodes
❑   H   is characterised histologically by keratin pearls

5.18 **Prognostic indicators for death from breast carcinoma include**

☐ A   vascular invasion
☐ B   presence of hyperchromatic nuclei
☐ C   negative excision margins for wide local excision
☐ D   presence of tubule formation
☐ E   oestrogen receptor status
☐ F   nodal status
☐ G   tumour grade
☐ H   tumour size
☐ I   presence of in situ carcinoma

5.19 **Gastric cancer**

☐ A   is a disease of affluence
☐ B   is more common in women
☐ C   has an increased incidence in patient's first-degree relatives
☐ D   is more common in individuals with blood group O
☐ E   has its highest annual mortality rate in China

5.20 **Factors associated with oesophageal cancer include**

☐ A   smoking
☐ B   Plummer-Vinson syndrome
☐ C   Barrett's metaplasia
☐ D   xeroderma pigmentosum
☐ E   pancreatic cancer
☐ F   achalasia
☐ G   peptic ulceration
☐ H   familial adenomatous polyposis

5.21 **The following tumours and corresponding serum markers are correctly paired:**

❑ A rectal carcinoma – carcinoembryonic antigen (CEA)
❑ B ovarian carcinoma – CA19-9
❑ C papillary carcinoma of the thyroid – calcitonin
❑ D testicular teratoma – alpha-fetoprotein
❑ E hepatocellular carcinoma – human chorionic gonadotrophin (hCG)
❑ F osteosarcoma – CA125

5.22 **Colorectal cancer**

❑ A occurs commonly in the autosomal recessive syndrome familial adenomatous polyposis
❑ B is the UK's third most common cancer
❑ C is common in vegetarians
❑ D accounts for 75% of all large bowel cancers
❑ E is caused by p53 gene mutations

5.23 ***Helicobacter pylori***

❑ A infects the stomachs of up to 25% of the world's population
❑ B is found submucosally in gastric biopsies
❑ C can be tested for serologically
❑ D detection kits exploit its secretion of dehydrogenase enzymes
❑ E can be eradicated by a week's treatment with clarithromycin and amoxycillin
❑ F is implicated in the pathogenesis of gastric lymphomas

5.24   Malignant melanoma

❑   A   is the most common cancer of young adults
❑   B   generally arises in a pre-existing naevus
❑   C   has its prognosis best predicted by Clark's levels
❑   D   lesions greater than 1.0 mm thick require a minimum 5 cm
            excision margin
❑   E   develops within lentigo maligna within 5–10 years

**5.25   Common carcinogens and their associated malignancies
            include**

❑   A   ultra violet radiation and basal cell carcinomas
❑   B   naphthylamine and gastric cancer
❑   C   asbestos and mesotheliomas
❑   D   benzene and colonic cancer
❑   E   arsenic and transitional cell carcinoma

5.26   Cancer registries

❑   A   would benefit from an increased hospital post-mortem rate
❑   B   are only useful for retrospective studies
❑   C   are most useful at a local level
❑   D   can monitor improved five year survival rates
❑   E   have no value in cancer screening

5.27   Hamartomas

❑   A   may be present at birth
❑   B   arise at the vermilion border of the lip in Peutz-Jeghers
            syndrome
❑   C   are mass lesions
❑   D   contain a variety of normal tissue components
❑   E   grow autonomously

5.28   Adenomas

☐ A   are typically encapsulated
☐ B   can arise in transitional epithelial cells
☐ C   exhibit cellular nuclear pleomorphism
☐ D   are typically annular lesions
☐ E   invade normal tissue

5.29   A $T_2N_1M_0$ tumour

☐ A   when applied to colorectal carcinoma is equivalent to a
          Dukes' B classification
☐ B   when applied to breast carcinoma is equivalent to Manchester
          stage II
☐ C   when applied to breast carcinoma indicates ipsilateral fixed
          axillary lymphadenopathy
☐ D   generally has a better prognosis than a $T_1N_2M_0$ tumour
☐ E   does not require adjuvant therapy

5.30   Dukes' staging of colorectal cancer

☐ A   is useful in determining the appropriate operative procedure
☐ B   is a valuable prognostic indicator
☐ C   defines a stage B as extending through the muscularis mucosa
☐ D   has regional lymph node involvement at stage C
☐ E   indicates an approximately 30% five year survival for those
          with stage C disease

5.31 Clinical features of bronchial carcinoma include

- ❑ A haemoptysis
- ❑ B hoarseness
- ❑ C ptosis
- ❑ D Sister Joseph's nodule
- ❑ E Sudeck's atrophy
- ❑ F polycythaemia
- ❑ G atrial fibrillation
- ❑ H pleural effusion

5.32 Typical features of a rectal carcinoma include

- ❑ A anaemia
- ❑ B constipation
- ❑ C melaena
- ❑ D mucous discharge
- ❑ E tenesmus

5.33 The following are appropriate applications of surgery to the management of malignant disease:

- ❑ A excision of a single enlarged inguinal lymph node after excision of a calf melanoma
- ❑ B latissimus dorsi flap reconstruction of a breast at the time of mastectomy
- ❑ C a left hemi-colectomy when liver metastases are found at laparotomy
- ❑ D a total gastrectomy when liver metastases are found at laparotomy
- ❑ E staging laparotomy and splenectomy for most patients with Hodgkin's disease
- ❑ F fixation of pathological femoral shaft fracture

5.34 Considering the use of CT scanning in malignant disease

- ❑ A 0.5 cm liver metastases are demonstrated
- ❑ B it clearly demonstrates pelvic recurrent disease
- ❑ C it is associated with minimal complications
- ❑ D it reliably assesses the suitability of a tumour to resection
- ❑ E it may be used after pacemaker insertion

5.35 Oncogenes

- ❑ A are normal cellular genes
- ❑ B in some cases encode growth factors
- ❑ C must be mutated to cause cancer development
- ❑ D exhibit a high degree of evolutionary variability
- ❑ E may be transmitted by viruses

5.36 Tumour suppressor genes

- ❑ A include p53
- ❑ B include the rhabdomyosarcoma gene
- ❑ C inhibit apoptosis
- ❑ D are commonly mutated in colonic cancer
- ❑ E mutations act in a recessive manner to induce neoplastic transformation
- ❑ F include genes encoding DNA-binding proteins which activate transcription

5.37 The ability of neoplastic cells to metastasise depends upon

- ❑ A tumour angiogenesis
- ❑ B decreased cellular cohesion
- ❑ C protease secretion
- ❑ D reduced cellular adherence to the basement membrane
- ❑ E increased production of cadherins

5.38   In the cell cycle

❑   A   DNA synthesis occurs during the M stage
❑   B   the cell is metabolically inactive in G_1
❑   C   the M stage leads to the production of two haploid cells
❑   D   changes in regulatory mechanisms may cause neoplastic
          transformation
❑   E   tissue growth rate depends on the length of the S phase

**5.39   In a histopathology report, the following terms are features of
          malignancy:**

❑   A   hypochromasia
❑   B   low nuclear to cytoplasmic ratio
❑   C   nuclear pleomorphism
❑   D   abnormal mitoses
❑   E   traverses the basement membrane

5.40   A screening test

❑   A   which is highly specific will have a low false positivity and
          high true positivity rate
❑   B   is only appropriate for a curable condition
❑   C   should have high sensitivity and low specificity for the disease
          in question
❑   D   for prostatic carcinoma is, ideally, PSA
❑   E   for colorectal cancer in high risk groups is, ideally, colonoscopy

5.41   Chemotherapy toxicity

❑   A   is reduced by combination chemotherapy
❑   B   may be increased in hepatic impairment
❑   C   may be treated by serotonin antagonists
❑   D   may be indicated by epistaxis
❑   E   may cause permanent hair loss

5.42   The following are useful tumour markers:

❑   A   alpha-fetoprotein and beta chorionic gonadotrophin in ovarian
            teratomas
❑   B   carcinoembryonic antigen in screening for colorectal cancers
❑   C   prostate specific antigen in monitoring prostatic carcinoma
❑   D   cancer antigen 125 in monitoring ovarian carcinoma
❑   E   alpha-fetoprotein in screening for hepatocellular carcinoma
❑   F   placental alkaline phosphatase

**5.43   The following hormone analogues are used in the treatment
             of malignancies:**

❑   A   octreotide
❑   B   pirenzepine
❑   C   goserelin
❑   D   cyproterone
❑   E   aminoglutethimide
❑   F   medroxyprogesterone acetate
❑   G   finasteride

5.44   Radiotherapy

❑   A   provides adjuvant treatment for squamous anal carcinoma
❑   B   is given post-operatively to improve survival in Dukes' C rectal
            cancers
❑   C   can improve regional control of oral cancers when given to
            cervical lymph nodes
❑   D   causes oxygen-independent DNA damage
❑   E   fractionation reduces damage to normal tissues without
            affecting tumour response rates

5.45   Early complications of radiotherapy may include

- ❑ A infertility
- ❑ B hypothyroidism
- ❑ C bone marrow failure
- ❑ D acute leukaemia
- ❑ E mouth ulcers
- ❑ F hair loss
- ❑ G diarrhoea
- ❑ H osteitis

5.46   Hypercalcaemia

- ❑ A may be a presentation of renal cell carcinoma
- ❑ B is a common feature of malignant disease
- ❑ C produces a positive Chvostek's sign
- ❑ D when not caused by hyperparathyroidism is most commonly due to malignant disease
- ❑ E may present with abdominal pain
- ❑ F may be a presentation of breast cancer
- ❑ G may be a presentation of colorectal cancer

5.47   The breast

- ❑ A lies between the 2nd and the 8th ribs
- ❑ B receives its blood supply exclusively from the internal and lateral thoracic arteries
- ❑ C overlies the external oblique muscle
- ❑ D lies directly on pectoralis major
- ❑ E has lymphatic drainage from the upper outer quadrants exclusively to the axillary nodes

5.48   The following are causes of gynaecomastia:

❑ A   bromocriptine
❑ B   cimetidine
❑ C   oral corticosteroids
❑ D   parathyroid gland tumours
❑ E   liver cirrhosis
❑ F   testicular teratomas
❑ G   adrenal gland tumour

5.49   In treating a breast abscess

❑ A   tetracycline is the antibiotic of choice
❑ B   aspiration may be successful
❑ C   breast feeding should be discontinued
❑ D   fistula formation is more common in smokers
❑ E   local anaesthetic must be used in pregnancy

5.50   Mammography

❑ A   when negative confirms that a breast lump does not need to be removed
❑ B   is superior to ultrasound in the detection of cysts
❑ C   detects significantly more tumours when two screening views are taken
❑ D   carries a small risk of inducing breast cancer
❑ E   is offered to all women over 50 years of age in the National Breast Cancer Screening Programme

5.51   The following are features of a fibroadenoma:

❑ A   cyclical changes
❑ B   most common in 30-40 year olds
❑ C   multiple
❑ D   fixed to skin
❑ E   spontaneously regress

5.52   Breast pain

☐   A   is common in the absence of sinister disease
☐   B   is not a symptom of cancer
☐   C   is most commonly non-cyclical
☐   D   may be due to Teitze's syndrome
☐   E   may be treated with tamoxifen

5.53   Fine needle aspiration cytology

☐   A   should be performed on all patients presenting with breast lumps
☐   B   should be performed prior to mammography
☐   C   should readily yield cellular material
☐   D   if acellular should always be repeated
☐   E   where cystic fluid is aspirated should always be sent for cytology

5.54   Fibroadenoma

☐   A   develop from single breast cells
☐   B   should be assessed by fine needle aspiration
☐   C   must be removed in patients over 40 years of age
☐   D   never develop into carcinoma
☐   E   bigger than 5 cm are known as phylloides tumours

5.55   The incidence of breast cancer is increased in

☐   A   atypical ductal hyperplasia
☐   B   late menarche
☐   C   late menopause
☐   D   oophorectomy
☐   E   obesity
☐   F   breast feeding
☐   G   nulliparity

5.56 Nipple discharge

- ❑ A is a feature of duct ectasia
- ❑ B occurs rarely in periductal mastitis
- ❑ C if bloody is diagnostic of malignancy
- ❑ D is always abnormal
- ❑ E will require total duct excision
- ❑ F is a common presentation of breast cancer

5.57 In the axilla

- ❑ A the axillary tail of the breast lies in the anterior wall
- ❑ B the mean number of lymph nodes is 35
- ❑ C the axillary vein lies medial to the artery and the cords of the brachial plexus
- ❑ D pectoralis minor muscle divides the axillary nodes into three levels
- ❑ E the intercostobrachial nerve is divided in axillary clearance

5.58 Wide local excision and axillary dissection

- ❑ A reduces psychological trauma in patients compared to those having mastectomy
- ❑ B requires supplementary radiotherapy to the breast for acceptable local disease control
- ❑ C histology should be checked for adequate resection margins
- ❑ D offers the advantage of staging axillary disease
- ❑ E is the preferred treatment for ductal carcinoma in-situ

5.59 Features of malignancy on mammograms include

- ❑ A spiculation
- ❑ B smooth margins
- ❑ C skin thickening
- ❑ D fine scattered microcalcification
- ❑ E encapsulation

5.60   Tamoxifen

❑   A   is an oestrogen receptor agonist
❑   B   adjuvant therapy for breast cancer should be continued for
ten years
❑   C   may be the sole therapy for breast cancer in the elderly
❑   D   is associated with an increased risk of endometrial carcinoma
❑   E   may produce menopausal symptoms
❑   F   may produce osteoporosis

5.61   Male breast cancer

❑   A   accounts for only 5% of all breast cancers
❑   B   treatment may require orchidectomy
❑   C   carries a worse prognosis than female breast cancer
❑   D   is associated with gynaecomastia
❑   E   is associated with a chromosomal abnormality

5.62   Palpable breast cysts

❑   A   may produce skin tethering
❑   B   are commonly bilateral
❑   C   are most common in the fourth decade
❑   D   should be re-aspirated each time they refill
❑   E   should be excised if they refill following aspiration
❑   F   usually contain blood-stained fluid

5.63   Paget's disease of the breast

❑   A   mimics psoriasis in the early stages
❑   B   is caused by intradermal infiltration by malignant cells
❑   C   is not invasive
❑   D   may lead to secondary sarcoma development
❑   E   is best treated by mastectomy and axillary clearance

5.64 **Routine investigations for a patient with radiologically and histologically confirmed breast cancer include**

❑ A chest X-ray
❑ B bone scan
❑ C liver ultrasound scan
❑ D CT scan
❑ E serum tumour marker levels

5.65 **A breast cancer can be differentiated from fat necrosis because of**

❑ A nipple retraction
❑ B mammographic characteristics
❑ C axillary lymphadenopathy
❑ D skin tethering
❑ E palpation of a discrete lump

5.66 **When managing screen detected breast lesions**

❑ A they should be excised and sent for frozen section to determine the best management
❑ B needle localisation facilitates excision
❑ C following excision the lesion should be sent for radiological assessment
❑ D the double-dye technique is better than the guide-wire/needle technique
❑ E excision is not always required

5.67   Breast reconstruction

❑ A   may use rectus abdominis or latissimus dorsi flaps
❑ B   may use a tissue expander to reduce the operative scarring
❑ C   can most simply be achieved with a prosthesis placed over pectoralis major muscle
❑ D   techniques may be used for salvage surgery
❑ E   myocutaneous flaps must not be given radiotherapy
❑ F   is contraindicated in the presence of DCIS

5.68   Adjuvant therapy for breast cancer includes

❑ A   tamoxifen in premenopausal women
❑ B   cyproterone
❑ C   tamoxifen in oestrogen receptor negative tumours
❑ D   ovarian ablation in premenopausal women
❑ E   combination chemotherapy in premenopausal women
❑ F   finasteride

5.69   In the UICC TNM classification of breast cancer

❑ A   a T_1 lesion should be < 2 cm
❑ B   a T_4 lesion should be > 5 cm
❑ C   an N_1 lesion has mobile ipsilateral axillary lymphadenopathy
❑ D   an N_3 lesion has fixed contralateral axillary lymphadenopathy
❑ E M_1 tumours would be Manchester stage IV

5.70   A patient with known metastatic breast carcinoma presents with vomiting. This may be due to

❑ A   opiate analgesia
❑ B   hypercalcaemia
❑ C   raised intracranial pressure
❑ D   gastric compression
❑ E   constipation

5.71   Pain relief in terminally ill cancer patients

- ❏ A   can always be achieved
- ❏ B   always requires the use of analgesics
- ❏ C   is given on an as required basis
- ❏ D   may be best given in the community by continuous subcutaneous infusion
- ❏ E   with opiates may improve respiratory problems

5.72   Common side-effects of opiates include

- ❏ A   nausea and vomiting
- ❏ B   dry mouth
- ❏ C   jaundice
- ❏ D   constipation
- ❏ E   confusion
- ❏ F   urinary retention

5.73   In terminal care bone pain may be reduced with

- ❏ A   radiotherapy
- ❏ B   NSAIDs
- ❏ C   prednisolone
- ❏ D   antidepressants
- ❏ E   TENS machine

5.74   Latissimus dorsi myocutaneous flap for breast reconstruction

- ❏ A   has a pedicle based on the thoracodorsal artery
- ❏ B   cannot be used for reconstruction following a subcutaneous mastectomy
- ❏ C   is not suitable for use with a synthetic breast prosthesis
- ❏ D   may be associated with post-operative contracture of the muscle
- ❏ E   may be associated with numbness of the axilla and upper inner arm

5.75   A palpable breast lump in a woman of 40 years

- ❑   A   is most likely to be a fibroadenoma
- ❑   B   should be investigated by ultrasound only
- ❑   C   investigated by mammography alone has a sensitivity for malignancy of 90%
- ❑   D   may be ductal carcinoma in situ
- ❑   E   may be associated with a positive paternal family history

5.76   The following drugs are ideal for continuous subcutaneous infusion in terminal care:

- ❑   A   morphine for analgesia
- ❑   B   methotrimeprazine for control of nausea and agitation
- ❑   C   hyoscine to reduce bronchial secretions
- ❑   D   amitryptyline for nerve pain
- ❑   E   domperidone for nausea and vomiting

5.77   Acute post-operative confusion may be caused by

- ❑   A   urinary tract infection
- ❑   B   hyponatraemia
- ❑   C   benzodiazepines
- ❑   D   hypovolaemia
- ❑   E   lower limb ischaemia
- ❑   F   hypoxia

5.78   Informed consent for a surgical procedure

- ❑   A   requires the patient to be informed about stomas prior to a right hemi-colectomy
- ❑   B   requires the patient to be informed about the risk of pancreatitis after ERCP
- ❑   C   is required for procedures under local anaesthetic
- ❑   D   requires the same information to be given to all patients
- ❑   E   is proved by a consent form

5.79   Gynaecomastia

❏   A   is usually unilateral
❏   B   is due to hypertrophy of the subcutaneous fat
❏   C   is usually self-limiting
❏   D   may be caused by cyproterone
❏   E   is usually treated with danazole

5.80   In a patient with nipple discharge

❏   A   galactorrhoea may be caused by hypoprolactinaemia
❏   B   blood stained discharge should always be investigated
❏   C   blood stained discharge is most commonly due to duct ectasia
❏   D   duct excision is favoured for multiple duct discharge

5.81   A patient brought in unconscious following a road traffic accident

❏   A   may have an emergency laparotomy without any consent if haemodynamically unstable
❏   B   may undergo procedures which the surgeon, acting as proxy, deems appropriate
❏   C   may have a blood transfusion
❏   D   may be placed on a ventilator with a view to organ donation
❏   E   may have blood taken for alcohol level measurement at the request of the police

5.82   Obtaining informed consent for a surgical procedure

❏   A   involves reference to a patient's moral rights
❏   B   involves respect for patient autonomy
❏   C   requires only that the patient signs a consent form after an explanation of the procedure
❏   D   is unnecessary in a patient detained under Section 3 of the Mental Health Act
❏   E   on children capable of expressing an opinion requires that their views be held paramount

5.83   It is mandatory for patient confidentiality to be breached

❑   A   at the request of a judge
❑   B   when a patient's criminal activities are suspected of posing a
           serious risk to others
❑   C   when a patient is known to be continuing to drive a car
           despite being medically unfit
❑   D   when a patient is suspected of terrorist activities
❑   E   when a patient has a notifiable disease

ANSWERS – CORE MODULE 1: PERIOPERATIVE MANAGEMENT 1

1.1 Suitability for day surgery   Answers: ABD

Day surgery patients should not be left alone for the first 24 hours after the procedure and they must have access to a telephone to summon assistance if required. Obesity (usually when the BMI is over 32 in day surgery) is a contraindication for day surgery because of the increased incidence of surgical and anaesthetic problems. The BMI is the weight in kg divided by the height in metres squared. Only ASA (American Society of Anesthesiologists) grade 1 and 2 patients are suitable. Insulin-controlled diabetes mellitus requires close monitoring of the glucose and therefore must be treated as an in-patient procedure. The protracted drainage after axillary clearance makes day surgery inadvisable.

1.2 Day surgery procedures   Answer: C

Patients undergoing day surgery only rarely require any premedication. Spinal anaesthesia makes mobility after surgery difficult. A caudal block is useful particularly with anorectal surgery. Femoral nerve blocks may make it difficult for the patient to walk. Anything that reduces patient mobility is a major disadvantage for day surgery. Drains can be used and are usually small suction drains that are removed prior to discharge or the next day by the community or general practice nurse.

1.3 Co-amoxiclav   Answers: ABD

Co-amoxiclav consists of amoxycillin and clavulanic acid (a β-lactamase inhibitor which inactivates penicillinases). Cholestatic jaundice is an adverse reaction occurring during or shortly after use. The risk of acute liver toxicity is six times greater than with amoxycillin. The treatment of systemic MRSA infection includes vancomycin or teicoplanin with colonisation being controlled by topical agents such as mupirocin.

1.4 *Clostridium tetani*   Answers: CE

Clostridium tetani produces protein exotoxins (tetanospasmin and tetanolysin) rather than endotoxins. It does not spread beyond the wound but the toxin is absorbed at the motor endings travelling to anterior horn cells of the spinal cord. If a wound is dirty, human derived anti-toxin should be given together with toxoid. The antitoxin provides passive immunity for four weeks. Gas gangrene is caused by *Clostridium perfringens*.

1.5   Acute response to Injury   **Answers: ACE**
In the acute phase of an injury the body starts a catabolic phase where
increased catecholamines cause glycogen to be broken down in the liver
and muscle to provide glucose. Insulin levels fall and the glucose levels
are raised. Increased sympathetic activity also causes mobilisation of fat
in adipose tissue.

1.6   *Bacteroides* species   **Answers: DE**
Bacteroides are Gram-negative, non-sporing, non-motile anaerobes
found in large numbers in the colon, genital tract and mouth. The most
common species is *Bacteroides fragilis* which is usually found with other
organisms, notably coliforms. Metronidazole and co-amoxiclav are both
effective against *Bacteroides* infections.

1.7   Scrubbing Up   **Answer: D**
Scrubbing up will not render the surgeon's hands sterile. One should aim
for socially acceptably clean hands. If anything, repeated washing
liberates more bacteria. The drying of hands is very important and
mechanical devices are no substitute for a sterile towel.

1.8   Acute alcohol withdrawal   **Answers: ABD**
Alcohol withdrawal (delirium tremens) can usually be predicted from a
properly taken history. It is characterised by agitation, overactivity,
disorientation and pyrexia. It leads to rapid dehydration and possibly
abdominal wound dehiscence. Adequate rehydration and correction of
metabolic alkalosis forms the basis of treatment together with diazepam
or chlormethiazole.

1.9   Sterilisation   **Answers: BCE**
Phenol and ethanol are only disinfectants and do not guarantee
eradication of spores or all bacteria. Buffered glutaraldehyde fluid is
used for endoscopes and requires at least 45–60 minutes' exposure.

1.10   Nutritional support   Answer: C

Multiple trauma causes a catabolic state and nutritional support is almost always required. The enteral route (either by fine bore nasogastric tube or percutaneous endoscopic gastrostomy) is preferred as this promotes intestinal blood flow and can reduce the incidence of stress ulceration. The parenteral route is associated with an increased incidence of complications such as catheter sepsis and problems related to catheter insertion. There are no studies which have shown a marked improvement in post-operative results with pre-operative feeding.

1.11   Pre-operative hypertension   Answers: ABCE

Longstanding untreated hypertension (systolic > 160 mmHg and diastolic > 110 mmHg) increases peri-operative morbidity and mortality and is a significant risk factor for coronary atherosclerosis. There is no association with DVT and PE. Sodium nitroprusside relaxes peripheral smooth muscle thereby reducing arterial blood pressure.

1.12   *Escherichia coli*   Answers: ABDE

Nosocomial means hospital-acquired. *E. coli* is a Gram-negative bacillus which can produce both endotoxin and exotoxin. It is a common cause of diarrhoea through its exotoxin. It is usually sensitive to cephalosporins, ciprofloxacin and aminoglycoside antibiotics.

1.13   Post-operative wound infection   Answers: ACEF

The non-microbial factors influencing the incidence of post-operative infection include dead/damaged tissue within a wound, excessive use of diathermy or mass ligature. Facemasks contribute little to prevention of wound infection. Excessive pressure or tension in the tissues may impair the circulation of both blood and lymph. Inadequate haemostasis results in 'dead space', haematoma or seroma formation providing a favourable nidus for bacterial growth. A well-controlled diabetes mellitus patient is no more susceptible to infection than the normal individual. Steroids and cyclosporin suppress the host's response to infection by depressing antibody function, diminishing phagocytic activity and inhibiting new capillary formation.

1.14   **Answer: B**

The use of pre-operative baths and shaving does not reduce infection rates. Nor is there any evidence that adhesive drapes reduce infection rates. Chlorhexidine is clear and has dye added to it to give colour to aid in delineating the completeness of skin preparation. An aqueous solution should be used in the perineum and if alcohol based preparation is used then care must be taken that it is allowed to dry and pooling is avoided.

1.15   **Human immunodeficiency virus (HIV)**   **Answer: C**

Occupationally acquired HIV infection in health workers occurs as a result of sharps injury, with hollow needles carrying a much greater risk. The overall risk of transmission of HIV infection is about 0.36% of all needle stick injuries in HIV-positive patients. There is no good evidence that post exposure chemoprophylaxis with zidovudine is effective. 6–12 weeks following HIV infection there is a rise in antigen titre but no detectable antibody. At three months 85% of HIV patients mount an antibody response and the antigen levels fall. In HIV infection the CD4 (receptors found on helper T cells and macrophages) count falls. Hepatitis B is thought to be over 1000 times more infective than HIV.

1.16   **Course of antibiotics**   **Answers: CD**

Antibiotics should be used to treat infection. Three doses are usually used for routine bowel surgery. Clean operations need no cover unless synthetic material is to be inserted (e.g. hernia repair with mesh). Localised abscesses do not respond to antibiotics because the abscess cavity is avascular and so the antibiotics cannot penetrate. Surgeons' views, however, vary on the use of antibiotics.

1.17   **General anaesthesia**   **Answers: AB**

The assessment and preparation of a patient is of vital importance. A family history would alert one to the possibility of suxamethonium sensitivity and malignant hyperpyrexia. It is important to omit oral hypoglycaemic agents before surgery, as hyperglycaemia is safer than hypoglycaemia. An ECG and chest X-ray should only be ordered if indicated. Premedication is not always required.

1.18   Opioids   Answers: BDE

Opiates act as receptors in the spinal cord and higher centres of the brain. Other routes of transmission include transdermal (fentanyl), sublingual (buprenorphine) and epidural.

1.19   Patient with COPD   Answers: ABC

The severity of chronic obstructive pulmonary disease can easily be assessed by how far the patient can walk without shortness of breath. The number of previous admissions to hospital related to the respiratory condition is important. $PaO_2 < 7.3$ kPa and $PaCO_2 > 6$kPa has a very poor prognosis and prolonged post-operative ventilation may be required.

1.20

A	cyst	3.	fluid filled tumour
B	papilloma	5.	overgrowth of epithelial tissue
C	plaque	1.	elevated area
D	macule	2.	flat lesion
E	hamartoma	4.	overgrowth of normal constituents

1.21   Metastasis   Answers: AC

Basal cell carcinoma or rodent ulcer advance locally, however, they do not metastasise. Lentigo maligna is a pre-malignant condition that, if left, will progress to a malignant melanoma in 10 to 30 years.

1.22   Patients with diabetes mellitus   Answers: ADE

Management depends on the magnitude of the operation and the severity of the diabetes. Patients with NIDDM require omission of their oral hypoglycaemic agents 48 hours before the operation. Post-operative observation is important with blood sugar, ketonuria and glycosuria. In the IDDM patient, an intravenous 5% dextrose drip is set up and the patient placed on an insulin sliding scale where the insulin infusion rate is adjusted on the basis of frequent blood glucose estimations.

1.23   Patient controlled analgesia   **Answers: ADE**
PCA usually contains an opioid such as morphine contained in a delivery system which will administer a preset bolus dose when the button is pressed by the patient. Fentanyl is too short acting and has marked respiratory depressant side-effects. The system has intrinsic safety features: bolus dose, lock-out interval, background infusion and maximum dose. PCA gives excellent analgesia comparable to epidural analgesia. It requires pulse oximetry monitoring but may cause respiratory depression on rare occasions.

1.24   Tourniquets   **Answers: BCE**
Tourniquets should not be applied for longer than 1.5 hours and the pressure should not exceed 300 mmHg. If the tourniquet needs to be used for longer, an interval of five minutes should be allowed before reapplying pressure. The most common effect on peripheral nerves is neuropraxia. Mechanical effects of compression and ischaemia cause focal demyelination. Axonotmesis means disruption of the axons while the nerve sheath remains intact.

1.25   Plain bupivacaine   **Answers: ABC**
Bupivacaine should not be used in a Bier's block because of marked cardiovascular depression that can occur after bolus i.v. injection. All local anaesthetics exhibit tachyphylaxis and cross the placenta. The maximum safe dose is 3 mg/kg. Tachyphylaxis is a process in which tolerance of the drug develops so that increasing doses are required to produce a particular effect.

1.26   Face masks   **Answers: BE**
Face masks provide very little protection. Few bacteria are dispersed from the mouth during quiet breathing and quiet conversation. Re-use leads to contamination as does wet 'strike through'. Disposable masks are made of synthetic fibres and contain filters of polyester and polypropylene. A new mask should be used for every procedure. Masks afford the wearer protection from 'splash' contamination.

1.27   Sterilisation by steam   Answers: BCI

Sterilisation by steam kills vegetative bacteria viruses and heat resistant spores such as *Clostridium perfringens*. It utilises a pre-set automatic cycle of steam under pressure, typically 134°C (30 lb/in^{-2}) for three minutes. Porous load autoclaves are checked daily using a steam penetration test (Bowie Dick) and cycle performance recorded as a temperature chart. Meshes used for inguinal hernia repair are sterilised by ethylene oxide.

1.28   Pulse oximeters   Answers: DE

Pulse oximeters monitor pulse rate, pulse volume and oxygen saturation. The oxygen saturation can be normal due to high inspired oxygen level. Pulse oximetry is accurate to 2%. Pulse amplitude is only an indicator of cardiac output. High concentration of carboxyhaemoglobin can cause a pulse oximeter to give a falsely elevated result. All colour changes are sensed, the change in path length caused by arterial pulsation allows subtraction of changes caused by capillary and venous blood.

1.29   Bipolar diathermy   Answer: D

Diathermy involves the passage of high frequency alternating current through the body. Bipolar diathermy avoids the need for a plate and uses considerably less power than monopolar diathermy. In bipolar diathermy, the current passes down one limb of the forceps through a small piece of tissue to be coagulated and then back to the generator via the other limb of the forceps. It is safe to use on appendages, such as fingers, toes, the pinna and the penis.

1.30   NdYAG laser   Answers: CDE

The NdYAG (Neodymium Yttrium Aluminium Garnet) laser penetrates tissue deeply (3–5 mm). It is useful for coagulating large tissue volumes, being especially useful in ablation of the exophytic part of an oesophageal carcinoma, controlling intestinal haemorrhage and treatment of low-grade bladder cancer. Safety measures are of paramount importance and a designated area with nominated users should be listed. Adequate eye protection is required at all times during laser procedures.

1.31   Wound infection   Answers: AD
Masks confer no proven benefit. Peritoneal lavage after a contamination reduces infection rates. The skin should be shaved as close to the time of surgery as possible or depilatory creams may be used. Closed suction drains reduce haematoma formation and so reduce wound infection but are not substitutes for meticulous haemostasis.

1.32   Gram-negative bacilli   Answers: BCDE
Bacterial meningitis is caused by cocci (*Neisseria meningitidis*). The intestine contains *E. coli, Klebsiella, Salmonella* and *Shigella,* all of which may cause food poisoning. *Pseudomonas aeruginosa* may cause a great number of problems on burns units in that it will interfere with skin grafting and carries a high mortality rate. *Haemophilus influenzae* is one of the most common causes of pneumonia in patients with chronic obstructive pulmonary disease. Liver abscesses are commonly due to *Streptococcus milleri*.

1.33   Commensal bacteria

A	cerebrospinal fluid	7.	sterile
B	colon	1.	*Bacteroides fragilis*
C	upper respiratory tract	3.	*Strep. viridans*
D	bile	7.	sterile
E	bladder	7.	sterile
F	stomach	7.	sterile

Cerebrospinal fluid, bile and urine should all be sterile under normal circumstances. The lower gut has many commensal organisms, *Bacteroides* being one. *Strep. viridan*s is a common upper respiratory tract commensal.

1.34   Wound infection rates   Answers: BCD
Any process such as poor retraction or over-tight suturing causes tissue trauma and ischaemia and therefore leads to necrosis, increasing the likelihood of wound infection. Other factors include concurrent illness, long pre-operative hospitalisation period, poor nutrition and immuno-suppression.

1.35   Fire hazards   Answers: ABE
A relative humidity of 60% is the lowest point at which surfaces will conduct away static charges. Resistance of articles should not be greater than 100 MΩ (to allow static dissipation) and not less than 0.5 MΩ (to protect against electrocution).

1.36   Day case surgery   Answer: D
Day case surgery is performed only by consultants or suitably experienced surgical trainees under supervision. Only ASA grades I and II are allowed (RCS criteria). The operating list should be confined to day cases so that there is less chance of cancellation due to bigger cases. Day case surgery is cheaper, as it reduces the need for an in-patient stay.

1.37   Staphylococci   Answers: BD
Staphylococci are Gram-positive aerobes that form grape-like clusters. Streptococci form strings and are grouped A to C.

1.38   Streptococci   Answers: ACD
Cellulitis is caused by these bacteria, usually group A (haemolytic type). *Strep. viridans* is a commensal in the throat and so need not be pathological. Staphylococci form bunches, Streptococci form strings.

1.39   Gram-positive rods   Answers: ACD
Diarrhoea can be caused by *Clostridium difficile* because of the development of pseudomembranous colitis. Tetanus is caused by toxins from *Clostridium tetani*. Not all Gram-positive rods are anaerobic.

1.40   Adequate renal function   Answer: B
Minimum urine output is 0.5 ml/kg/hr in a normal adult representing 30 ml/hr or more. The urine osmolality should rise after fluid depletion, indicating that the kidneys are concentrating urine. A normal MSU does not show that the kidneys are working adequately, however, an abnormal MSU may indicate the converse. A diuresis does not show that the kidneys are functioning well, as the urine may be of very poor quality with a low osmolality as in the diuretic phase of renal failure.

1.41   T-tubes   **Answers: CDE**

T-tubes are used to drain the common bile duct after exploration. They produce a controlled fistula to protect against the sinister effects of a bile collection. They are removed at ten days after surgery if a T-tube cholangiogram demonstrates that there is no distal obstruction, there is free flow of contrast into the duodenum and there are no retained stones. The drains are made of latex rubber, which causes an intense reaction, and so forms a controlled fistula to the skin. This facilitates external drainage of bile after the removal of the tube. ERCP and sphincterotomy have reduced the incidence of intraoperative common bile duct exploration. The drain should be brought out through a separate hole to reduce the risk of wound infection.

1.42   Abscess   **Answers: ABC**

The white count is not necessarily raised, but this is a common feature. The patient will have a fluctuant swelling. Induration may indicate an abscess is too deep to demonstrate signs of fluctuance, whilst a chronic discharge will be due to a fistula.

1.43   Drains for surgical procedures

A	thyroidectomy	3.	suction
B	primary inguinal hernia repair	5.	none
C	total hip replacement	3.	suction
D	perforated appendix	4.	tube drain
E	anterior resection	4.	tube drain
F	perforated duodenal ulcer	5.	none
G	subphrenic abscess	1.	sump
H	right hemicolectomy	5.	none
I	axillary clearance	3.	suction

The traditional view is that cervical surgery such as thyroid and parathyroid surgery requires the use of a suction drain to avoid respiratory complications of haemorrhage. Corrugated drains are ideal for the drainage of a contaminated wound, leaving the skin loosely approximated. The use of drains after colonic anastomosis is in dispute. However, if a drain is to be used then a large closed tube system is indicated although corrugated drains can also be used. Sump drains are useful when there is a large abscess cavity in the abdomen or pelvis, because tissue is less likely to block the drain holes in a sump drain. There is a general trend away from corrugated drains towards closed systems because of the risk of transmission of infection to ward staff.

1.44   Drug adverse reactions

A	atenolol	4.	bronchospasm
B	cisplatin	2.	nephrotoxicity
C	glyceryl trinitrate	1.	hypotension
D	NSAID	3.	peptic ulceration

1.45   Organisms

A	*H. influenzae*	4.	pneumonia
B	*E. coli*	1.	urinary tract infections
C	*Candida albicans*	2.	oesophagitis
D	*Proteus*	1.	urinary tract infections
E	*Staph. aureus*	5.	wound infection
F	*Strep. milleri*	6.	liver abscess

1.46   Anaemic patients   Answers: CD
Optimal haemoglobin level is a compromise between oxygen carrying capacity and viscosity with the optimum haemoglobin being 10 g/dl. There is some evidence that perioperative transfusion may cause transient immunosuppression and so increase recurrence rates for colonic tumours. Oral iron should increase the haemoglobin 1 g/dl/wk. Large transfusions the day prior to surgery cause problems because the oxygen carrying capacity is reduced while the 2,3 diphospho-glycerate in the stored blood is replenished.

1.47   Intravascular coagulopathy   Answers: BC
The platelet count is usually much lower than this due to consumption leading to a raised INR (international normalised ratio) and also raised fibrinogen degradation products due to intravascular lysis of the clotting components. Surgery may be the only treatment that can correct the cause of DIC and so is not contraindicated. However, the clotting must be corrected as much as possible beforehand with platelet transfusion and fresh frozen plasma. GMCSF (granulocyte macrophage colony stimulating factor) is used in leucopenia.

1.48   Steroids   Answers: AE
Steroids may cause Cushing's syndrome with bruising, striae, centripetal weight gain, a buffalo hump and moon face. They may also raise mood (especially useful in terminal care) and cause hirsutism.

1.49   Lung disease
Answers: ACDF

Stopping smoking even one day prior to surgery improves outcome by reducing the blood carbon-monoxide levels. Pre-operative ventilation will only increase the chance of a lower respiratory infection. Respiratory stimulants such as doxapram have no role. Unless the patient has a chest infection, antibiotics have little to add.

1.50   Diagnosis of breast disease
Answers: ABCE

Contrast studies may be used to look at breast ducts in a ductogram. CT scanning is useful in the investigation of metastases but not the primary disease. Doppler may be used in conjunction with ultrasound to look at the vascularity of a lump, however, duplex scanning is not used. Impedance tomography is an experimental technique of no proven value. Radionuclide imaging is useful in the management of metastatic malignancy. MRI may have a particular role in differentiating a fibrous scar from recurrence after surgery for breast cancer.

1.51   Magnetic resonance imaging
Answers: AF

MRI is a very good imaging technique for examining the musculoskeletal system (particularly the knee and vertebral column) and for anorectal and pelvic disease. In may be used in conjunction with paramagnetic contrast agents such as gadolinium. Some patients cannot tolerate the procedure due to claustrophobia and patients with metal implants cannot be imaged due to the strong magnetic fields used.

1.52   Abdominal surgery in a diabetic patient
Answers: CD

Only type 1 (IDDM) diabetics have a general anaesthetic. Type 2 (NIDDM) diabetics having major surgery require a sliding scale and should be first on the list. An ECG is required because of the high risk of cardiac disease which may be symptomless. Chlorpropamide has a long half-life and so should be stopped the day before surgery or an investigation requiring intravenous contrast.

1.53   NSAIDS with an acute abdomen
Answers: BC

A plain abdominal X-ray in an acute abdomen in a patient of this age, without the features of bowel obstruction, is unlikely to be helpful. However, an erect chest film will show free gas from a perforated duodenal ulcer in 70% of cases and a left lateral decubitus film may be helpful. Ultrasound is seldom helpful unless it is thought the patient may have cholecystitis or pancreatitis.

1.54   Chest X-ray   Answers: BCDE
Patients over 50 years old with a concurrent history of hypertension or
smoking should have a chest X-ray. Immigrants from countries with a risk
of TB should have a chest X-ray.

1.55   Polyglactin sutures   Answers: All false
Polyglactin ('Vicryl™') sutures are absorbable but take months to absorb.
They cause little tissue reaction compared with biological sutures.
Vicryl™ is usually braided and not suitable for vascular anastomosis
because of its lack of strength and its absorption.

1.56   Biological sutures   Answers: ABE
Biological sutures (such as silk), due to their braided nature, are
associated with the formation of sinuses and when they were used for
vascular anastomosis caused false aneurysms. Their breakdown is
unpredictable, therefore, synthetic sutures have many advantages.

1.57   Mass abdominal closure   Answers: CD
Mass closure should follow Jenkins' rule of 4:1. The most important layer
is the anterior sheath. Remember that the posterior sheath is deficient
below the arcuate line. Goodsall's rule applies to anal fistulae. PDS and
Dexon, which are absorbable sutures, are used in mass abdominal
closure.

1.58   Pre-operative blood count   Answers: BDE
For all except major surgery, young fit children and fit adults do not
require a full blood count unless there is a risk of missing unsuspected
disease such a thalassaemias and haemoglobinopathies in those of Afro-
Caribbean origin or because of other medical problems.

1.59   ECG prior to surgery   Answers: BCDE
All patients over 60 should have an ECG as should any patient with a
history of hypertension, peripheral vascular disease or ischaemic heart
disease. Patients having vascular operations or those that involve
thoracotomy should all have ECGs irrespective of whether they are
symptomatic or not.

1.60   Keloid scars   **Answers: AE**
Keloid scars extend beyond the previous wound (hypertrophic scars are confined to the wound). They are most common on the sternum and the deltoid area, usually re-excision leads to a recurrence unless steroids are locally injected to reduce the scar formation. Pressure dressings work well but the use of subcuticular sutures is of no value.

1.61   Skin excision margins   **Answers: CD**
Squamous carcinomas should be excised with a 1 cm margin and basal cell carcinomas with a 0.5 cm margin. The advised margin for a melanoma depends upon the depth of invasion of the lesion. For impalpable lesions 1 cm is sufficient, while for a nodular lesion the margin should be 3 cm. The margin required depends on the Breslow thickness, but this can only be determined by examination of a biopsy specimen. The external appearance may give some guide as to the excision margin required.

1.62   Diathermy   **Answers: ADE**
Diathermy uses high frequency current 400 kHz to 10 MHz, the high frequency prevents electrocution. The coagulation setting has a sine wave with a frequency of about 15 kHz, whereas cutting uses a more continuous power output in a square wave. Due to the wave types the energy distribution pattern is different causing more tissue vaporisation on cutting and more protein denaturation and coagulation on this setting.

1.63   Lasers   **Answers: ABE**
Laser or Light Amplification by the Stimulated Emission of Radiation produces high power coherent beams of monochromatic light. The energy is in the form of photons. Not all medical lasers are invisible although many are and need an aiming light. Argon beam lasers are blue-green.

1.64   Anaesthesia   **Answers: BCDE**
Ketamine is used with cardiac disease, as it is one of the few agents that does not suppress the myocardium. Propofol has a rapid onset and relatively rapid recovery time and so is often used for day case surgery.

1.65   Anaesthetic and the ventilated patient   Answers: BDEH
The minimum monitoring includes assessment of airway pressures, pulse oximetry and end tidal CO_2 along with the ECG. Constant arterial blood gases are not routinely taken except for major surgery such as cardiac surgery.

1.66   Local anaesthetic agents   Answers: DE
Local anaesthetic agents block sodium channels in nerves, the first affected are the small non-myelinated fibres (c fibres), this is why motor impulses are preserved despite anaesthesia. The active state of the agents is the anionic one and this is why the action of local agents is dependent on pH. They do show tachyphylaxis, which is the need for an ever-increasing dose due to acquired tolerance.

1.67   Maximum safe doses   Answers: ABDE
A 1% solution contains 10mg in 1ml of solution. The safe doses are:

	Plain	With adrenaline
Lignocaine	3	6
Bupivacaine	2	2
Prilocaine	7	–

Doses in mg/kg. Prilocaine with adrenaline is not used.

1.68   Intravenous injection of local anaesthetic   Answers: BDC
Circumoral tingling is the classical first sign of inadvertent intravenous injection of local anaesthetic agent. This then may lead to cardiac tachyarrhythmias and convulsions and eventually coma and death.

1.69   Deep vein thrombosis   Answers: ABCEFGH
The risk of deep vein thrombosis is increased when any of Virchow's triad (blood flow changes, blood composition change or vein wall trauma) are altered and thereby increase the propensity for the blood to coagulate.

1.70   Routine DVT prophlaxis   Answers: BCDE
Full anti-coagulation is not needed routinely, although it may be necessary for a patient with an increased risk of thrombosis. Graduated elastic stockings (e.g. TED™ (thromboembolism deterrent) stockings) are widely used. Good hydration of the patient is essential.

1.71   Spinal anaesthesia   Answer: A
Spinal injection is a relatively short-lived anaesthetic and cannot be topped up in the post-operative period in contrast with epidural anaesthesia. Spinal injection may also cause a lowering of the blood pressure due to vasodilatation and so the patient must be well filled prior to its injection. A dural tap may cause a headache.

1.72   Brachial plexus block   Answers: BCDEG
The usual route of administration is interscalene however suprascapular and direct axillary routes are also used. This method may be used for pre- and post-operative analgesia for surgery on the arms. A catheter may be inserted in an epidural.

1.73   Epidural analgesia   Answers: ABCEFG
Severe liver damage is associated with disorders of coagulation making epidural anaesthesia hazardous. Due to the drop in blood pressure after epidural injection of local anaesthetic agents, they are contraindicated in shock and sepsis. Multiple sclerosis can be exacerbated by epidural analgesia and so this should also be avoided. Far from being contra-indicated, epidurals are used frequently in obstetrics.

1.74   General anaesthesia   Answers: BCDE
Pre-emptive analgesia is the term used for giving analgesics prior to pain to prevent the sensation from starting. This in turn reduces the absolute analgesic requirement. As the name implies this pre-empts the situation. Benzodiazepines have no innate analgesic action.

1.75   Sedation   Answers: ABCDE
Any patient with a reduced ability to maintain their airway and with increased response or unpredictable response to sedation is especially at risk.

1.76   Biopsy   **Answer: B**

Biopsy of testicular neoplasm is rarely needed because the diagnosis can usually be based on clinical examination and ultrasound. Cold-cup biopsy forceps can be passed down the working channel of the side-viewing endoscope at ERCP to biopsy bile duct lesions. Needle biopsy is more appropriate for muscle tumours because of the risk of dissemination. Full-thickness biopsies are required to make a diagnosis of Hirschsprung's disease because it is not a mucosal disease but aganglionosis of the muscle layer.

1.77   Fasting   **Answers: BCD**

A patient should be starved for any operation where there is a possibility of the need to convert to a general anaesthetic or the use of concurrent sedation. The general rule is that food should not be taken for six hours prior to surgery and liquids for four hours. However, sips and normal medication can be taken up to the time of surgery.

1.78   Bier's block   **Answers: CD**

When any form of regional analgesia is used, resuscitation facilities should be at hand including a tilting trolley and oxygen. A cardiac monitor is not essential but should be available. Flumazenil is a benzodiazepine antagonist and is not used. Bupivacaine should never be used for a Bier's block due to its cardiac toxicity, bearing in mind that the tourniquet may fail allowing access to the general circulation and that there is intra-osseous flow through the humerus.

1.79   Adrenaline with local anaesthetics   **Answers: ABD**

Adrenaline has many advantages when used in conjunction with local anaesthesia. It reduces bleeding and the absorption of the agent and so potentiates the effect and makes surgery easier. By slowing absorption it allows a larger total dose of agent to be used. It should never be used in a ring block due to the possibility of digital artery spasm and consequent ischaemia.

ANSWERS – CORE MODULE 2: PERIOPERATIVE MANAGEMENT 2

2.1 **Patient undergoing a right hemi-colectomy** **Answer: A**
Steroids are known to delay wound healing and patients who have had long-term doses will require parenteral treatment during the post-operative period to prevent Addisonian crises.

2.2 **Wound repair** **Answers: ACDE**
Following injury, coagulation forms the first step, activating complement and platelet aggregation. The inflammatory phase peaks at 12 hours post injury. Matrix remodelling commences after 24 hours whereby extracellular matrix is synthesised and degradation occurs.

2.3 **Healing following sigmoid colectomy** **Answers: ACDEF**
To promote good anastomotic healing there must be no tension, good blood supply and no infection. Steroids, malignancy, vitamin C deficiency, zinc deficiency, diabetes mellitus and jaundice are all thought to inhibit normal wound healing.

2.4 **Haemacel** **Answers: BCDE**
The normal CVP range is 3–8 cm H_2O. A low or negative reading confirms a low circulating blood volume. The response of the CVP to a fluid challenge of colloid gives much information regarding the state of the circulation. A dehydrated patient's CVP will rise in response to a challenge but fall to the original value as the circulation vasodilates. A sustained rise indicates a well-filled patient but an elevation of greater than 4 cm H_2O indicates overfilling or a failing myocardium.

2.5 **Haemacel** **Answer: C**
Haemacel is a solution of degraded gelatin and contains ten times more calcium (6.25 mmol/l) and potassium (5.1 mmol/l) than gelofusin. The half-life of haemacel is five hours. Hespan is a 6% solution of hydroxyethyl starch in 0.9% saline. Dextran 70 affects the coagulation system by inhibiting platelet aggregation and renders fibrinogen more susceptible to fibrinolysis.

2.6   Pulmonary aspiration   Answers: ABCE
This is a serious complication carrying a high morbidity and mortality. Minor degrees of aspiration are common. Massive aspiration occurs either during induction and intubation or during recovery from general anaesthesia. Treatment includes bronchial tree suction toilet, antibiotics and bronchodilators. IPPV may be required. Rapid sequence induction anaesthesia is essential. Antacids and an H_2-receptor agonist are used in obstetric anaesthesia to reduce effects of aspiration pneumonia (Mendelsohn's syndrome).

2.7   Answers: ACD
A 70 kg man is approximately 70% water, having a fluid volume of about 49 litres. This is divided into the intracellular and extracellular spaces in a ratio of 2:1. The extracellular fluid is further divided into 12 litres of interstitial fluid and 3 litres plasma. Fluid is normally lost in the form of urine (1500 ml), through the skin (900 ml), in expired air (400 ml) and in the faeces (200 ml). The normal daily requirement of nitrogen is 15 g/day.

2.8   Fresh frozen plasma (FFP)   Answers: BCD
FFP is prepared by freezing plasma to -30°C within six hours of collection. It can be stored for up to twelve months. If there is a delay in administration once it has thawed, the coagulation factors (especially factors V and VIII) lose their activity. FFP should be ABO and rhesus compatible. It should not be used to correct hypovolaemia, as it is wasteful of valuable clotting factors.

2.9   Side-effects of cyclosporin   Answers: ACE
Other complications include; nephrotoxicity, hepatotoxicity, hyper-tension, tremor and haemolytic anaemia.

2.10   Immune response reduction   Answers: ACD
HIV infection per se will not cause immunosuppression. However after seroconversion the disease AIDS will cause it.

2.11   Organ transplantation   **Answers: BCD**
The HLA is carried on the short arm of chromosome 6. The class 1 antigens are A, C, B, and the class 2 include DR, DP, DQ. The matching of graft and recipient relies on the leucocyte reaction test. It would appear that the DR antigens may be more important than the A,B antigens.

2.12   Side-effects of steroids   **Answers: ABD**
Other side-effects include diabetes, Cushing's syndrome, obesity and cataracts. Azathioprine causes polycythaemia, hepatotoxicity and bone marrow suppression.

2.13   Wound healing   **Answers: ABE**
Wound healing is dependent upon systemic factors and local ones. Systemic factors include adequate nutrition including vitamins C, A and zinc. Steroids have an inhibitory effect on healing. Excessive movement or the presence of foreign bodies in the wound also delay healing. The wound must also have an adequate blood supply.

2.14   Anastomotic leak   **Answers: ABDE**
Septic shock may be the first sign of a leak. The patient may also develop a distended abdomen and pass pus or diarrhoea. A leak may be confirmed by a contrast enema avoiding the use of barium, but should always be suspected when the patient is not recovering in the expected way, as the signs and symptoms may be non-specific.

2.15   Peripheral vein parenteral nutrition   **Answers: BCDE**
PPN is considered safer than central vein TPN. The solutions in PPN have a lower osmolality. Suitable peripheral veins are required, the main limitation is the hypertonicity of solutions. GTN, low dose heparin and hydrocortisone in the infusion may prolong the infusion site life.

2.16

A	thyroidectomy	3.	none
B	hernia repair	4.	non adherent
C	incision and drainage abscess	2.	alginate ribbon
D	varicose vein avulsions	1.	pressure dressing
E	haemorrhoidectomy	5.	paraffin ribbon

Many dressings are available. The alginate dressings have the advantage of being haemostatic and also desloughing.

2.17   Haemophilia A   **Answer: B**
Haemophilia A is a sex-linked coagulation disorder characterised by low or absent factor VIII clotting activity. The bleeding time is normal and epistaxis is not as common as it is in thrombocytopenia. Blood stored at 4°C quickly loses factor VIII activity and therefore it should be isolated from fresh blood.

2.18   Incompatible blood transfusion   **Answers: ABEG**
Most transfusion reactions are haemolytic in nature. Chest pain and paraesthesia are sometimes seen in the early stages. Haemoglobinuria, haemoglobinaemia, oliguria and jaundice occur relatively late. Myoglobinuria occurs as a result of muscle destruction.

2.19

A	Yates	5.	tube open
B	Wallace/Robinson	3.	closed tube
C	corrugated	2.	open
D	Redivac	1.	closed vacuum
E	sump	4.	irrigating

Drainage systems are defined as open or closed (to the open air). Sterility is best maintained with a closed system and so they are used for sterile collections. The closed systems can be dependent or under a vacuum. For heavily contaminated areas, an open non-tube drain is best as this is less likely to occlude.

2.20   Subclavian vein cannulation   Answers: CD
The subclavian route is associated with an increased number of complications such as pneumothorax. It is inserted by Seldinger technique – inserting the needle below the clavicle at the junction between the middle and outer two-thirds of the clavicle.

2.21   Low molecular weight heparin   Answers: BC
LMWH (4000–5000 Daltons) preferentially neutralises activated factor X, a key factor in the promotion of thrombin generation. Unlike standard unfractionated heparin, which is highly negatively charged, it is not neutralised by platelet factor 4. It has excellent bioavailability and has a longer half life than heparin. Due to the favourable pharmacology of LMWH, no laboratory monitoring is required.

2.22

A	hernia wound	3.	primary closure
B	abscess drainage incision	2.	secondary intention
C	abdominal wound post faeculant peritonitis	5.	delayed primary closure
D	burns to face	4.	excision and grafting
E	circumferential burns	1.	escharotomy

Escharotomy involves cutting through the full thickness of a burn in order to relieve a constriction due to the burnt tissue or eschar. In burns some are best treated by immediate excision and split skin grafting.

2.23   Post-operative retention of urine   Answers: ABCD
Post-operative retention of urine is far more common in men than women due to benign prostatic hypertrophy. It is a common cause of post-operative abdominal pain/discomfort, especially following haemorrhoidectomy. The treatment is bladder catheterisation (urethral or suprapubic). Finasteride is used to treat benign prostatic hyperplasia in the long term. Bethanechol is an anticholinergic drug which may precipitate retention.

2.24   Nutritional support   Answers: DE

Patients on enteral nutrition have a lower incidence of pneumonia and wound infection compared with those having parenteral nutrition. Enteral nutrition maintains the gut mucosal barrier and may prevent bacterial translocation which may lead to multi-organ failure. Peripheral parenteral nutrition is not recommended for longer than two weeks as there is a high risk of thrombophlebitis, thrombosis and line infection. In addition, the calorific content of peripheral parenteral nutrition is not as high as TPN. The metabolic complications of TPN include hyperglycaemia, hypokalaemia and vitamin and trace element deficiency.

2.25   5% dextrose intravenous infusion   Answer: A

5% dextrose becomes hypotonic as the dextrose is metabolised. It is evenly distributed through all the fluid compartments and only a small amount stays within the intravascular space. Type I respiratory failure may be caused by infusion of 5% dextrose which contains 30 kcal and 278 mmol glucose per litre.

2.26   Complications of burns   Answers: ACD

Major burns are associated with many complications in keeping with other major trauma. Muscle loss can lead to myoglobin in the urine which together with hypovolaemic shock causes renal failure. The patient may become low in Na^+ due to water toxicity.

2.27   Autologous blood   Answers: AC

Autologous blood transfusion eliminates the transmission of infectious disease. It is indicated for fit patients between the ages of 18–65 years who have no cardiac, respiratory or cerebral disease. Blood should not be collected in the presence of infection. Up to four units may be collected over a four week period with the last collection four days before the operation.

2.28   Glomerular filtration rate (GFR)   Answers: AC

GFR varies in life. Adult levels are reached at 2 years of age and decline linearly from 40 years of age due to glomerular sclerosis. It is measured by insulin clearance, but clinically measured by creatinine clearance. A 50% increase in GFR occurs during pregnancy. GFR increases after a protein rich meal.

2.29   Metabolic acidosis   Answers: CDF

Metabolic acidosis is the result of accumulation of any acid other than carbonic acid or the loss of bicarbonate. Increased lactic acid production occurs when cellular respiration is abnormal resulting from either a lack of oxygen (type A) or metabolic abnormality (type B). Type A lactic acidosis is the most common acidosis seen in clinical practice occurring in septicaemia or cardiogenic shock.

2.30   Respiratory acidosis   Answers: ABE

Respiratory acidosis occurs when the $PaCO_2$ exceeds 7 kPa and is caused by hypoventilation. The causes can be divided into airway obstruction, intrinsic lung disease, neuromuscular problems, chest wall problems and central respiratory drive depression. Pulmonary embolus classically causes a respiratory alkalosis due to hyperventilation.

2.31   Hyponatraemia   Answers: BDE

Excess steroids lead to hypernatraemia and hypokalaemia due to activation of the sodium/potassium pump in the distal convoluted tubule. Pyrexia leads to water loss and hence hypernatraemia. Burns cause loss of sodium from wounds. Irrigation following TURP may lead to excessive water absorption (the TUR syndrome).

2.32   Head injuries with a skull fracture   Answer: A

An isolated head injury with no skull fracture but a reduced Glasgow Coma Scale has a 1/120 chance of a significant intra-cranial injury. This is raised to 1/4 with a skull fracture. If the patient has a normal GCS and a fracture then the risk is 1/32.

Alcohol in itself does not necessitate a CT scan of the head, however if there is a reduced conscious level then one cannot assume that it is solely due to intoxication.

2.33   DIC   Answers: ABC

DIC occurs secondary to other disease processes such as trauma, burns or sepsis. It arises from intravascular activation of procoagulant factors, chiefly thrombin and platelet aggregation or adhesion leading to widespread thrombosis of microcirculation of several organs. Treatment is directed to the causes and replacement of clotting factors is essential.

2.34 von Willebrand's disease   Answers: BCE

von Willebrand's disease is inherited in an autosomal dominant fashion caused by a deficiency of vWF factor. There is a prolongation of bleeding time and APTT but a normal PT time. It is characterised by bleeding from skin and mucous membranes and, unlike haemophilia A, haemarthroses are rare. In type I von Willebrand's disease, infusion of desmopressin (d-desaminoarginine vasopressin – 'DDAVP') will increase factor VIII and vWF and is used to cover minor surgical procedures.

2.35 Cardiac contusion following trauma   Answers: ACE

In major trauma a cardiac contusion may be associated with other chest injuries. The features are ECG changes of ischaemia (T wave tenting is due to hyperkalaemia). The creatinine kinase will be raised in all significant trauma and so only the isoenzyme assay will be of use.

2.36

A	oral Co-proxamol	3.	circumcision
B	epidural catheter	1.	caesarian section
C	20 ml 1% local anaesthetic	2.	hernia repair
D	75 mg intramuscular pethidine	5.	pancreatitis
E	patient controlled analgesia	4.	left hemi-colectomy

2.37 Blood testing   Answers: ACEG

Currently in the United Kingdom, microbiological screening includes hepatitis B surface antigen and antibodies to syphilis, HIV 1 and 2, and hepatitis C. A few cases of hepatitis B transmission occur each year through carriers with undetectable hepatitis B surface antigen.

2.38 Complications of blood transfusions   Answers: ACDE

Metabolic acidosis may occur due to increased amount of lactic acid in stored blood. Hypothermia occurs as a result of rapid infusion of large quantities of cold banked blood which may itself exacerbate acidosis and further impair the mechanism of coagulation. Hypocalcaemia is related to transfused citrate in banked blood. Stored blood has few platelets and may result in a dilutional thrombocytopenia.

2.39   Raised MCV   Answers: AE
A raised MCV is seen in vitamin B_{12} and folate deficiency as well as alcohol abuse and paraproteinaemia. A reduced MCV is seen in thalassemia and iron deficiency and the anaemia in renal failure is either microcytic or normocytic.

2.40   Post-operative pain relief   Answers: DE
Oral analgesics are rarely helpful in the initial analgesia of post-laparotomy patients. These patients are often 'nil by mouth' and also will have delayed gastric emptying. Patient Controlled Analgesia (PCA) uses a continuous infusion of morphine and antiemetic. Fentanyl is far more potent than morphine having greater respiratory depressant side-effects. It does, however, have a very short half-life. These should be used under controlled circumstances with close monitoring. Bupivacaine has the longest duration of action. However, it is the most toxic of the available local anaesthetic drugs, the main toxicity is that on the myocardium.

2.41   Sickle cell disease   Answers: BDE
Vaso-occlusive sickling in SCD causes bony avascular necrosis, acute splenic sequestration, hypersplenism, priapism often causing impotence, leg ulcers and peripheral sickle retinopathy (PSR). PSR relates directly to an increased risk of vitreous haemorrhage and retinal detachment. Excessive haemolysis causes gallstones which should, ideally, be removed. The acute chest syndrome is the main post-operative cause of morbidity and mortality. It is characterised by fever, leucocytosis, chest pain and lung consolidation.

2.42   Sickle cell disease   Answers: BD
SCD often presents with an acute abdominal crisis. There are sickle cells, target cells and Howell-Jolly bodies (suggesting splenic atrophy) in the peripheral blood. SCD is due to a substitution of valine for glutamic acid in position 6 on the fl-chain. There is no normal HbA detectable. The amount of HbF varies from 5–15%.

2.43   Prolonged irrigation   Answers: ABCD
Absorption of irrigating fluids during irrigation can lead to so-called TURP syndrome, causing a metabolic acidosis, hyponatraemia and confusion and haemolysis.

2.44   Classification of surgical wounds

A	inguinal hernia repair	1.	clean
B	perforated diverticular disease with paracolic abscess	4.	dirty
C	laparoscopic cholecystectomy	2.	potential contamination
D	pilonidal abscess	4.	dirty
E	thyroidectomy	1.	clean
F	peritonitis from recent duodenal ulcer	4.	dirty
G	tracheostomy	1.	clean

3.1

A	blood loss 1.3 litre	4.	pale colour
B	blood loss 1.7 litre	3.	reduced systolic pressure
C	blood loss 2.5 litre	2.	unconscious
D	blood loss 0.75 litre	1.	normal heart rate
E	blood loss 1 litre	5.	raised diastolic pressure

Blood loss				
Litres	0.75	0.8–1.5	1.5–2.0	> 2.0
%	< 15%	15 – 30%	30% – 40%	> 40%
Blood pressure				
Systolic	Normal	Normal	Reduced	Very low
Diastolic	Normal	Raised	Reduced	Very low
Pulse	< 100	100–120	120 reduced vol	> 120 thready
Capillary refill	Normal	> 2 s	> 2 s	Nil
Respiratory rate	Normal	Normal	>20 bpm	>20 bpm
Urinary flow rate ml/h	> 30	20–30	10–20	< 10
Skin colour	Normal	Pale	Pale	Pale/Cold
Mental state	Alert	Anxious	Drowsy	Unconscious

3.2   Tension pneumothorax   Answers: CDE

In a tension pneumothorax the mediastinum is shifted away from the affected side. Breath sounds are reduced/absent and the chest is hyper-resonant.

3.3 Chest trauma
Answers: BCDE

Cullen's sign is peri-umbilical bruising due to retro-peritoneal bleeding. Rib fractures can be very well treated with analgesia either by a local block or a catheter in conjunction with oral analgesics, this enables effective physiotherapy which is vital to avoid infective complications. Flail segment needs no surgical treatment although some surgeons fix the fractures, they may however require the patient to be ventilated.

3.4 Burns
Answers: BD

Burns result in substantial loss of fluid, protein and blood. Many regimes calculating plasma replacement have been described including the Muir & Barclay formula. The requirement (ml/period) = Surface area burnt (%) x wt (kg)/2. In burns over 30% there is a higher incidence of ARDS, ileus and stress ulceration. Crystalloids should be avoided and cultures of urine, blood, wound, skin and sputum are used to identify the organism. Injudicious use of antibiotics leads to colonisation of resistant bacteria.

3.5 Staff in a major incident
Answers: ACE

During a major incident the organisation and distribution of labour is a key element. A communications centre should be set up comprising a senior nurse, a senior administrator and the A&E consultant. A senior clinician should perform the triage of the patients. A radiologist in the department aids greatly in the assessment of X-ray requests and interpretation. The junior staff may well be asked to 'act up' for more senior colleagues.

3.6 Nasotracheal intubation
Answers: ABD

Nasotracheal intubation can provide a definitive airway and is a useful technique when a cervical spine fracture is confirmed or suspected or when urgency of the airway management precludes a cervical spine X-ray. Nasotracheal intubation is contraindicated in the apnoeic patient, severe mid-face fractures or suspicion of base of skull fracture. It may be used in the conscious patient using local anaesthetic spray.

**3.7   Measurements on lateral cervical   Answers: All false
         spine films**

When examining a lateral cervical spine film, in addition to inspecting for obvious fractures, the depth of prevertebral space should be assessed to look for evidence of soft tissue swelling associated with a fracture, the predental space should be measured to look for any evidence of atlantoaxial instability and the relative heights of the anterior and posterior borders of vertebrae assessed to look for evidence of crush fracture. The following are generally accepted as the upper limits of normal for adults:

A   ≤ 3 mm
B   < 2 mm
C   ≤ 7 mm
D   ≤ 22 mm (or the depth of the vertebral body)
E   > 13 mm

3.8   Features indicating major trauma   Answers: BE

A fall of more than 15 feet is associated with a significant probability of sustaining a major trauma, as is an extrication time of > 20 minutes or a vehicular impact speed > 30 mph (> 25 mph with no restraints). In addition a pedestrian impact with a car travelling > 20 mph is associated with significant risk of injury.

**3.9   Airway management of multiply injured   Answers: ABD
         patient**

Spontaneous breathing is a pre-requisite for nasotracheal intubation, a laryngoscope is not used, the tube is advanced as the operator listens to breathing sounds through the tube. No tube should be passed into the nose when there is clinical evidence of either facial fractures or a base of skull fracture as the tube could pass through into the brain. In trauma, oxygen must be given through a mask with a reservoir bag at 12–15 litres per minute, nasal prongs are not sufficient. Either needle or open cricothyroidotomy is indicated when endotracheal intubation has failed. The airway must be managed with the neck in in-line immobilisation until it has been cleared radiologically. The neck must not be extended to open the airway.

3.10   Peripheral nerves   Answers: BD

Peripheral nerves are usually mixed containing sensory fibres to the posterior root ganglia and afferent motor fibres from the anterior horn cells. The vasomotor fibres are also carried in the nerves. Pressure causes tingling after 15 minutes, neurapraxia is by definition reversible.

3.11   Nerve damage   Answers: ADE

In axonotmesis the nerve is disrupted usually by increased pressure or crushing. The axon sheath and endoneurium remain intact but the nerve distally and a little retrogradely is resorbed by Wallerian degeneration which takes a few days.

3.12   Neurotmesis   Answers: BCD

Neurotmesis describes total division of a nerve or the damage that occurs in severe traction injuries, crushing injuries and intra-neural injections. The nerve is resorbed but is replaced with scar tissue. Neuromata occur and recovery is never total.

3.13   Adult basic life support   Answers: All false

When coming upon a potential victim of cardiac arrest, the rescuer should check for responsiveness, if the victim is not responsive, help should be sought. The rescuer should check whether the victim is breathing by looking, listening and feeling for breaths for 10 seconds. If the victim is not breathing and help has not already been sought, then the rescuer should go immediately for help, before initiating resuscitation. On returning, up to five breaths should be given to attempt to achieve two effective breaths (an effective breath is one that makes the chest rise). The presence of a circulation should be checked for by looking for any movement and/or checking for a carotid pulse for up to 10 seconds. If there is no evidence for a circulation at 10 seconds, CPR should be commenced. The heel of the hand should be placed over the lower half of the sternum, the other hand should be placed on top. Compressions should commence at a rate of approximately 100 per minute to a depth of approximately 4–5 cm. The ratio for a single rescuer is 15 compressions to 2 breaths, for two rescuers 5 compressions to 1 breath.

3.14   Management of airway in children   Answers: CDE

Children have a relatively larger head which tends to flex the head on the neck, making airway obstruction more likely. The relatively larger tongue tends to flop back and obstruct the airway in the obtunded child and gives less room in the mouth when intubating. The larynx is more cephalically placed (glottis at C3 in infants compared with C6 in adults) and the angle of the jaw is larger in children (1400 in infants, 1200 in adults), both making intubation more difficult. In addition the trachea is shorter, and the cricoid ring is the narrowest part of the airway (compared with the glottis in the adult).

3.15   Resuscitation for multisystem trauma   Answers: BCD

To achieve the recommended FiO_2 of 0.85 supplementary oxygen should be administered via a face mask and reservoir bag. Type-specific uncrossmatched blood is preferred for transfusion as this reduces subsequent cross-matching problems. Urinary catheterisation is contra-indicated by blood at the meatus, blood in the scrotum or a high riding or impalpable prostate. Catheterisation may proceed after a urethrogram has confirmed continuity of the urethra. Cardiac arrhythmias (atrial fibrillation, premature ventricular contractions, ST changes) may indicate cardiac contusion, electromechanical dissociation may indicate tamponade, tension pneumothorax or profound hypovolaemia or hypothermia. The shock-like state associated with trauma is most often due to hypovolaemia and should be treated with vigorous intravenous fluid therapy.

3.16   Motorcyclist accident   Answers: ACD

In trauma, shock must be assumed to be haemorrhagic until proven otherwise. In this case the blood pressure is low but there is no extreme tachycardia. It is possible that this patient is a trained athlete who has a resting pulse of 40. In this case a pulse of 80 would be a relative tachycardia. Also, in late Class IV shock the pulse rate will drop as a pre-terminal event. Anaesthetic drugs, particularly Diprivan (propofol) can cause hypotension. Septic shock can follow a perforated viscus or contaminated wound, however this would not become manifest for several hours at the earliest. An extradural haematoma under pressure will cause a bradycardia and hypertension (Cushing's response).

3.17 Tachycardia in response to haemorrhage   Answers: ACE

Tachycardia in response to haemorrhage may be absent in the elderly, patients on beta-blockers and calcium antagonists, in hypothermia and in patients who have a pacemaker. Infants will develop a tachycardia but the rate will be much higher than in adults. Athletes have a higher blood volume, a higher cardiac output, a higher stroke volume and a lower resting pulse than the rest of the population. The usual responses to hypovolaemia may not be manifest in athletes, even though significant blood loss may have occurred. Oxygen will not affect this response.

3.18 Brachial plexus injuries   Answers: BE

Erb's palsy occurs in upper root lesions (C5,6 +/- 7) and Klumpke's palsy with lower ones (C8, T1). Erb's gives a 'waiter's tip' hand position whilst Klumpke's gives a claw hand. Sympathetic disruption is more common with lower lesions as the sympathetic fibres come from the T1 root. Post-ganglionic injuries may recover or be amenable to repair, preganglionic injuries are irreparable.

3.19 Damage to nerves   Answers: CE

Damage to the long thoracic nerve causes winging of the scapula, spinal accessory nerve damage will cause weakness on abduction of the arm. The axillary nerve contains fibres of C5, C6 nerve roots to supply predominantly the deltoid muscle with some sensory fibres to the lateral aspect of the forearm. Froment's sign is associated with ulnar nerve injuries where abductor pollicis is weak and so flexor pollicis longus accommodates.

3.20 Healing of fractures   Answers: DE

The first stage of any fracture healing is the formation of a haematoma. There then follows an intense inflammatory response where there is both cellular proliferation and also resorption. In this way woven bone is formed which then consolidates to form lamellar bone. This is then remodelled.

3.21 Non-union of fractures   Answers: BCE

Excessive movement will also cause non-union. Non-union can be either hypertrophic or atrophic. In hypertrophic non-union excessive amounts of useless callus is formed. In atrophic non-union very little callus is formed.

3.22 Internal fixation   Answers: BCE

Internal fixation will not lead to faster healing but it will give stability to the bone. If large opposite forces are present then splinting is unlikely to be successful and so fixation is needed. In the multiply injured patient internal fixation may reduce the incidence of complications. Internal fixation should be avoided in compound fractures due to the risk of infection.

3.23 Subdural haemorrhage   Answers: BCDE

Subdural bleeds are usually due to tearing of the bridging veins in the arachnoid layer. They are more common in babies, the elderly and alcoholics. These three groups share the fact that the subdural space is relatively larger than in the younger adult.

3.24 Glasgow Coma Scale   Answers: BD

Eye opening			Verbal response		
	none	1		none	1
	to pain	2		sounds	2
	to speech	3		words	3
	spontaneous	4		confused	4
				orientated	5

Motor response		
	none	1
	extension	2
	flexion	3
	withdrawal	4
	localise	5
	obey commands	6

3.25 Fractures   Answers: BCD

Petrous fractures of the skull are associated with V, VII and VIII cranial nerve palsies and not III N. With a skull fracture on plain X-ray there is a 1/32 chance of intra-cranial injury with a normal GCS, if this is reduced then the chance increases to 1/4.

3.26   Surgical airway   Answers: ACE
A surgical airway is indicated where there is the inability to intubate the trachea and when there is an immediate need for an airway. Insertion of a needle through the cricothyroid membrane is a useful technique in emergency situations to provide oxygen on a short term basis. A surgical cricothyroidotomy is performed by making a skin incision through the cricothyroid membrane and inserting a small endotracheal/tracheostomy tube (5–7 mm).

3.27   Blood loss   Answers: BD
This patient has lost approximately 20% of his blood volume. Clinical symptoms include tachycardia, tachypnoea (usually 20–30 breaths/min) and a decrease in pulse pressure due to elevation of diastolic blood pressure caused by a rise in catecholamines producing an increase in peripheral resistance. The systolic pressure does not change. Significant changes in mental status occur when there is greater than 30% volume loss (Class III or IV haemorrhage). Greater than 50% blood loss results in loss of consciousness.

3.28   Resuscitation fluids   Answers: CD
Normal saline contains 150 mmol/litre of sodium and chloride. Hartmann's solution contains 131 mmol/litre sodium, 111 mmol/litre chloride, 5 mmol/litre potassium and lactate. Gelofusine contains < 1 mmol/litre calcium and can be safely infused with blood (Haemacel contains 12.5 mmol/litre calcium and should be infused through a different line or be infused through a flushed line), both are derived from gelatin. Pentastarch has a duration of action of 7 hours, albumin 6 hours and Gelofusine and Haemacel 3 hours. Dextrose should not be used as a resuscitation fluid because of its short duration of action in the circulation.

3.29   Early response to trauma   Answers: CE
In the immediate aftermath of a traumatic insult to the body, a complex series of responses are set in motion. Underperfusion of the tissues leads to a decrease in metabolic rate and body temperature, and an increase in anaerobic metabolism with the formation of lactic acid and a secondary metabolic acidosis. Increased levels of catecholamines stimulate lipolysis and glycogenolysis which leads to hyperglycaemia in the presence of decreased insulin levels, this hyperglycaemia is exacerbated by the conversion of lactic acid in the liver to glucose.

3.30   Stabbing victim   **Answers: AB**
Distended neck veins are likely to be present in both a cardiac tamponade and in a tension pneumothorax. Air entry will be absent on the affected side, there will be hyper-resonance to percussion and the trachea will be deviated to the opposite side in a tension pneumothorax. The diagnosis of both conditions is clinical and time should not be wasted on any investigations. The treatment of a cardiac tamponade is immediate needle pericardiocentesis. The treatment of a tension pneumothorax is an immediate needle thoracocentesis to the affected side. A cannula is inserted into the second intercostal space in the mid-clavicular line. A central venous pressure reading is likely to be high in both conditions. Thoracotomy is not indicated in the immediate management in the case described here.

3.31   Subarachnoid haemorrhage   **Answers: BC**
SAH is characterised by the onset of the 'worst headache ever'. The blood can be easily identified on non-contrast CT in 90% in the first 48 hours. Trauma is the most common cause, aneurysms are responsible for 75–80% of spontaneous causes, AV malformations for 5% and the remaining 15% of spontaneous causes have unknown aetiology. Treatment involves control of BP, anti-epileptic medication, prevention of vasospasm with the calcium channel blocker nimodipine, and treatment of raised ICP. An angiogram is obligatory to rule out aneurysm. In patients with aneurysm, 20% will have multiple aneurysms. Early surgery (48–72 hours) is favoured in patients in good medical and neurological condition, with blood causing a mass effect. Delayed surgery (10–14 days) is favoured for patients in poor medical and neurological condition, and those experiencing effects of vasospasm.

3.32   Haemorrhage due to trauma   **Answers: ABDE**
Hypovolaemia is poorly tolerated in the elderly. Aggressive therapy with fluids is often warranted to prevent serious complications such as MI and CVA. The fit individual compensates very well for hypovolaemia as their stroke volume can increase by 50% with no increase in pulse rate. Beta adrenergic blocking agents and calcium antagonists may mask and alter the patient's haemodynamic response to haemorrhage.

3.33   Skull fractures   Answers: AB
Prophylactic antibiotics are only needed in skull fractures if there is an associated CSF leak from the nose or ears indicating a breach in the dura. If this is present then intubation of the stomach or trachea will increase the risk of meningitis. CSF is sterile and has no commensal bacteria. The commonest bacteria in post-fracture meningitis are from the upper respiratory tract.

3.34   Intraosseous infusion   Answers: DE
This procedure is limited to children six years or younger in whom venous access is impossible due to circulatory collapse or for whom percutaneous peripheral venous cannulation has failed on two attempts. The puncture site is on the anteromedial surface of the proximal tibia 1–3 cm below the tubercle. The Seldinger technique is one of needle puncture followed by the insertion of a guide wire. Over this a larger cannula can be inserted.

3.35   Skull X-ray after head injury   Answers: ABCD
After head injury, indications for skull X rays are:
* patients who are difficult to assess i.e. children, post-ictal epileptics, those with alcohol or drug intoxication
* patients with large scalp lacerations or contusions, particularly over the temporal region
* post injury seizure
* patients with abnormal neurological signs
* a reduced level of consciousness
* post traumatic amnesia.

Previous craniotomy, by itself is not an indication for skull X-ray after head injury.

3.36   Acute spinal cord transection   Answers: BDE
Apnoea ensues if the cord lesion is above C3. Injury involving C4–C6 results in insufficient tidal volume, progressive hypoxia and CO_2 retention. Lesions above T5 eliminate much of the sympathetic nervous system and ensuing vasomotor tone is low causing hypotension. Tachycardia is a compensatory response to hypotension.

3.37 Peripheral venous cutdown — Answers: CD

Peripheral vein cutdown is used for volume replacement when normal peripheral access is not possible. The surface marking for the greater saphenous vein is anterior and superior to the lateral malleolus.

3.38 Tension pneumothorax — Answers: ACE

A tension pneumothorax causes a shift of the trachea to the opposite side. It should be suspected if a patient has dilated neck veins, absent breath sounds and a hyper-resonant chest on the affected side. It should be diagnosed clinically and a needle/cannula should be inserted into the pleural space in the second intercostal space, mid-clavicular line as one cannot wait for the chest X-ray to be performed. The definitive procedure is to insert a chest drain connected to underwater seal drainage. A cardiac tamponade should be suspected when the heart sounds are muffled and when there are small complexes on the ECG.

3.39 Brain death — Answer: A

Brain death is caused by tissue hypoxia in the brain or hypoglycaemia. Hypoxia may occur due to lack of oxygenation or lack of perfusion; (hypotension or raised intra-cranial pressure). For a diagnosis the patient must fulfil the following:

i)   not under any central depressant or blocking drugs,
ii) core temperature above 35°C
iii) all metabolic disturbance corrected
iv) a cause established.

The following reflexes must all be absent and tests performed by two independent doctors of five or more years post qualification:
i)   pupillary and corneal
ii) vestibulo-ocular
iii) gag reflex
iv) doll's eye reflex
v)   absent ventilatory effort despite full oxygenation (FiO$_2$ 100%) and a rising pCO$_2$ on the withdrawal of ventilatory support.

3.40   Spinal injury   Answers: ADE
The most common site of injury is the cervical spine. Urinary or faecal incontinence is always of significance. Spinal injuries may mask abdominal or chest injuries due to anaesthesia. The triage priorities are as always airway, breathing and circulation in that order. (Spinal injuries are of little consequence if the patient is not breathing or has no blood pressure.)

3.41   Chest trauma   Answers: AE
Massive haemothorax may be difficult to see on chest films and great volumes of blood may be lost before it is apparent. Most bleeds will stop after the insertion of a chest tube and adequate fluid resuscitation and few need exploration. The diagnosis of tension pneumothorax is a clinical and not radiological one and exerts its main effect via reducing cardiac return and so causing circulatory compromise.

3.42   Major accident plan   Answers: BCDE
Major accident plan for the oncall surgeon includes reporting to the triage/charge person.

3.43   Revised Trauma Score   Answers: BDE
The Revised Trauma Score is compiled using coded values for respirarory rate, systolic blood pressure and the Glasgow Coma Score.

Parameter	Value	Coded value
Respiratory rate	10–29	4
	>29	3
	6–9	2
	1–5	1
	0	0
Systolic blood pressure	>90	4
	76–89	3
	50–75	2
	1–49	1
	0	0
Glasgow Coma Score	13–15	4
	9–12	3
	6–8	2
	4–5	1
	3	0

3.44   Injury severity scale   Answers: ABC

The Abbreviated Injury Scale ranges from 1 (minor) to 6 (fatal). There are six designated regions of the body used for calculating Injury Severity Score; head and neck, abdomen and pelvic contents, bony pelvis and limbs, face, chest and body surface. An Injury Severity Score of > 16 is taken to indicate major trauma, the maximum obtainable Injury Severity Score is 75 ($5^2+5^2+5^2=75$), a single Abbreviated Injury Scale score of 6 in any single region is automatically given an Injury Severity Score of 75.

3.45   Split thickness skin grafts   Answers: CDE

Split skin grafts are commonly used to repair clean, vascularised, non-infected wounds or granulation tissue. Relatively avascular sites (e.g. bone without periosteum or irradiated wounds) are not capable of nourishing a graft. Split skin grafts are totally separated from their blood supply and adhere to the recipient bed by fibrinogen deposition. Required nutrients are obtained by diffusion – oxygen and nutrients diffuse well through plasma but not through blood clot. Split skin grafts do not require direct pressure although this can help to reduce seroma or haematoma formation. However, grafts must be immobilised, notoriously difficult in some areas (e.g. the back).

3.46   Maxillofacial trauma   Answers: AE

Le Fort fractures
I)   low maxillary fractures only, cause malocclusion
II)   as above with extent into the infra-orbital rim and nasal area
III)   separation of the mid face from the cranium

Tracheostomy is a formal operation and should be carried out in controlled circumstances in the operating theatre, a cricothyroidotomy may be carried out as an emergency.

3.47   Answers: AC

The skull is thickest at the occiput and base. The most exterior layer is the dura mater which is a tough fibrous sheath. The next layer is the arachnoid mater which transmits the nutrient vessels to the brain. Applied to the brain surface is the thin pia mater. The CSF is external to the pia and internal to the dura.

3.48 Aortic rupture   Answers: AEF

Aortic rupture is suggested by a widened mediastinum (i.e. > 8 cm) which is the most reliable finding. Obliteration of the aortic knuckle, elevation and rightward shift of the right main-stem bronchus, depression of the left main-stem bronchus and presence of a pleural cap are the other features that may be seen on the chest X-ray.

3.49 Traumatic diaphragmatic hernia   Answers: ACE

Diaphragmatic rupture is uncommon. It may occur following both penetrating and blunt trauma to the chest or abdomen. A stomach or intestinal gas pattern is commonly seen in the left hemithorax. A nasogastric tube is both diagnostic and therapeutic. Other diagnostic aids include a barium swallow or pneumoperitoneum.

3.50 Diagnostic peritoneal lavage   Answers: BC

Diagnostic peritoneal lavage should be performed in the multiple injured patient if the abdominal examination is equivocal, unreliable or impractical. It is 98% sensitive for intraperitoneal bleeding. The only absolute contraindication is an existing indication for laparotomy. Relative contraindications include previous abdominal operations, morbid obesity, advanced cirrhosis and pre-existing coagulopathy. A positive test is indicated by 100,000 RBCs/mm^3 or >500 WBC/mm^3 in the fluid aspirated from the peritoneum after instilling 1 litre of saline infra-peritoneally.

3.51 Acute extradural haematoma   Answers: BCFG

Acute extradural haematoma almost always occurs from a tear in a dural artery, usually the middle meningeal artery. A small percentage occur as a result of a tear in the dural sinus. Acute extradural haematoma occurs in only 0.5% of unselected head injuries. The signs and symptoms include loss of consciousness followed by an intervening lucid interval then development of hemiparesis on the opposite side and a fixed dilated pupil on the same side. The mortality is nearly zero in the non-comatose patient and 20% in deep coma.

3.52 Fractures of tubular bones   Answers: ACE

Cell proliferation at the fracture site occurs early. The callus at the fracture site is usually profuse in children because the periosteum is easily stripped from bone by extravasated blood.

3.53   Complications of fractures   Answers: AC

The incidence of myositis ossificans, commonly seen at the elbow, is increased by open operation. Late rupture of extensor pollicis longus as it rubs over Lister's tubercle is classically seen in Colles' fracture of the wrist. Damage to the radial nerve as it winds round the back of the humerus may produce wrist drop in some fractures of the shaft of the humerus. Paraesthesia is a late sign of compartment syndrome, increasing pain, a tense compartment and pain on passive flexion are earlier signs. Classically the peroneal nerve is damaged in tibial plateau fractures.

3.54   Compartment syndrome   Answers: ACDE

Compartment syndrome is the term used to describe the condition in which the tissue pressure in an enclosed fascial compartment rises above the capillary pressure thus reducing blood flow to the distal tissues. The early signs include paraesthesia (complete anaesthesia is a late sign), pink shiny skin, pain in the affected muscles on passive stretching and a feeling of pressure. Distal pulses and capillary refill may be present even in the presence of significant increases in compartmental pressure. Although direct measurement of compartmental pressures can be made, the condition is often treated on clinical grounds, with removal of any occlusive dressings and elevation followed by fasciotomy if needed.

3.55   Compartment syndrome   Answer: E

'High-risk' injuries for compartment syndrome include fractures of the elbow, the radius and ulna and proximal third of tibia. The presence of a pulse does not exclude compartment syndrome. If there is diagnostic doubt, compartment pressures can be measured. If > 40 mmHg (with a normal diastolic pressure), immediate fasciotomy is required.

3.56   Cervical cord injury   Answers: ACD

Cervical cord injury is characterised by flaccid areflexia, diaphragmatic breathing, ability to flex but not extend the elbow. Priapism is an uncommon but characteristic sign. Full immobilisation of the neck is required at all times.

3.57   Maxillofacial trauma   Answers: CDE
The most common cause of maxillo-facial trauma is assault since the introduction of seat belts. Hooding of the eye is associated with Le Fort III fracture due to detachment of the facial skeleton from the skull base. The contents of the superior orbital fissure may be damaged if the fracture line runs along the orbit.

3.58   Following trauma   Answers: ACDE
Following trauma, there is an elevation of ADH, catecholamines and cortico steroids that have the effect of conserving water and producing a hyperglycaemia.

3.59   Cerebro-spinal fluid   Answers: AC
Cerebro-spinal fluid is produced predominantly in the ventricles which are connected via the foramen of Monro. The CSF is produced at a rate of 0.3–0.5 ml/hr. The arachnoid villi are involved in the re-absorption of CSF into the venous sinuses and so into the systemic circulation.

3.60   Cerebral blood flow   Answers: BD
Cerebral perfusion pressure is calculated by the mean arterial blood pressure minus the intracranial pressure; it is under strict autoregulation and so in the normal subject fluctuates very little despite many postural changes. The autoregulatory stimuli are pO_2 and pH (pCO_2 has its effect via the dissociation to HCO_3^- and H^+ ions and so fall in pH). Mannitol is used to reduce intracranial oedema and so reduce intracranial pressure in the pathological state, increasing blood flow, but there is no increase in normal subjects.

3.61   Extra-dural haemorrhage   Answers: ABD
The injury is either to the middle meningeal artery or to the dural venous sinuses. In the majority of patients the ipsilateral pupil dilates with contralateral motor signs; this is due to pressure on the temporal lobe affecting the III nerve.

4.1 Bronchiectasis   Answers: ACDE

Childhood infection may cause destruction of the alveoli and dynamic closing of the relatively non-cartilaginous bronchi, which in turn leads to progressive dilatation and mucus gland hypertrophy. Kartagener's syndrome is where there is a congenital deficiency of cilia, which then causes secretion build up (as in cystic fibrosis). Treatment is largely that of physiotherapy and treating infections. Resection may be indicated for unilateral disease, which is fairly well localised.

4.2 Intermittent Positive Pressure Ventilation (IPPV)   Answers: AF

IPPV alters the distribution of ventilation and perfusion in the lung and increases venous admixture and perfusion in the lung. Lung compliance remains unchanged or may fall if a low tidal volume is used.

4.3 Functional Residual Capacity (FRC)   Answers: ACDE

FRC represents the volume of the lungs at the end of a normal tidal breath. It is reduced intraoperatively because of increased activity of muscles of respiration and elevation of the diaphragm. Pain and splinting of the diaphragm occur post-operatively in abdominal surgery. With age there is loss of elastic tissue and hence FRC rises.

4.4 Oxygen-haemoglobin dissociation curve   Answers: ADE

The oxygen-haemoglobin dissociation curve is shifted to the right by a fall in pH, pyrexia, 2,3-DPG elevation and pCO_2 rise which all help to dissociate oxygen from haemoglobin. Carbon monoxide combines with haemoglobin to form carboxyhaemoglobin, reducing the total capacity of blood to carry oxygen.

4.5 Pulmonary embolism   Answers: CDF

Pulmonary embolism causes hypoxia and hypocapnia due to hyperventilation. The most common ECG change is a sinus tachycardia, there may be features of right ventricular strain with right bundle branch block. Spiral CT may be of use to diagnose proximal segmental emboli. A mismatch on V/Q scan confirms the diagnosis. Tinzaparin is a LMWH (Low Molecular Weight Heparin) licensed for the treatment of pulmonary embolism.

4.6   Superior mediastinum   Answers: ABE
The superior mediastinum lies above the level of T4 and so contains all the above except the right main bronchus which arises below this level. The heart forms the middle mediastinum.

4.7   Lung sepsis   Answers: ACE
The treatment of an empyema is surgical drainage. For a chronic infection an open procedure will be needed. At this time the lung will have a thickened cortex over its surface which will need to be removed to clear the infection. Decortication and open drainage rarely cause trouble from persistent pneumothorax. Antibiotics are the treatment of choice in an abscess. These rarely need percutaneous drainage.

4.8   Intercostal drain   Answers: BDE
An intercostal drain should be inserted in the 5th intercostal space in the mid axillary line and so should not penetrate pectoralis. The visceral pleura overlies the lung and should not be entered, although this may inadvertently occur.

4.9   The right ventricle   Answers: BD
The right ventricle is the most anterior. Although it is the most likely of these chambers to be penetrated in sharp trauma to the chest, this is still improbable. Being anterior it is best visualised by standard echo. It is supplied by the right coronary artery and receives blood from the bronchial veins (remember the dual circulation of the lungs).

4.10   Dissection of the ascending aorta   Answers: BCD
Dissection of the ascending aorta (Debakey type I and III) may disrupt the ostia of the coronary arteries and so cause cardiac ischaemia and infarction. Distortion of the aortic valve may occur leading to valvular incompetence. Rupture into the pericardium can cause tamponade, but this is rare.

4.11   Left coronary artery   Answers: CDE
The right marginal and the sinu atrial artery are both branches of the right coronary artery.

4.12   Atrial fibrillation   **Answers: BCDE**

Atrial fibrillation is associated with, but does not cause, mitral valve disease. However, it may lead to thrombus forming in the enlarged atria and so lead to emboli causing stroke, gangrene of either digits, limbs or even the bowel. Dyspnoea may be due to left ventricular failure as a result of too rapid a heart rate or rate dependent ischaemia or infarction.

4.13   Auscultation of the heart

A   left anterior axillary line second intercostal space   5. none
B   apex   1. mitral valve
C   5th intercostal space mid clavicular line   1. mitral valve
D   left sternal edge 2nd intercostal space   4. pulmonary
                                                                 valve
E   right sternal edge 5th intercostal space   3. tricuspid
                                                                 valve

4.14   Central line insertion   **Answers: ABDE**

4.15   Inotropic effect on the heart   **Answers: BCE**

Dopamine at low doses has an effect on pure dopaminergic receptors, only at higher doses it has a truly inotropic effect via β receptors. Calcium and digoxin (the first inotrope) are both inotropes. Frusemide may have an inotropic effect if used to offload a failing ventricle, but is in itself not inotropic.

4.16   Shock   **Answers: BCD**

The initial treatment of hypovolaemic shock is obviously fluid replacement, the same is true for septic shock although antibiotics and vasopressor agents should also be used. In anaphylactic shock vasoconstrictors should be used first, but fluid replacement will also have a role. Cardiogenic shock needs inotropic support and possibly off loading and so fluids would only worsen the situation. Obstructive shock caused by tamponade or pulmonary embolism needs drainage or vasodilators respectively.

4.17   Insertion of central venous catheter   **Answers: ABCDF**

All of the above complications can occur together with the inadvertent cannulation of an artery, with the exception of stroke.

4.18   Jugular venous pressure (JVP)   **Answer: B**
The JVP is increased in cardiogenic and obstructive shock. No waves are
evident in atrial fibrillation and with the patient flat then the JVP is full.
This is the position for measuring central venous pressure via a central
line. A CPAP (constant positive airway pressure) ventilation causes
delayed venous return and so raises the JVP.

4.19   Pulmonary artery flotation catheter   Answers: EF
Pulmonary artery flotation catheters directly measure cardiac output by
a thermal dilution technique (modified Fick principle). They also
measure directly the CVP, wedge pressure, mean blood pressure and
mean pulmonary artery pressure. This allows calculation of systemic and
pulmonary vascular resistance.

4.20   Coronary circulation   Answers: BC
Coronary circulation occurs during diastole (systole causes occlusion of
the coronary arteries lumens). The arteries are end arteries; this is why
the heart infarcts in a specific distribution. Autoregulation does occur in
a supply and demand fashion by the release of metabolites such as
adenosine. The circulation does not reverse and 5 l/min is the average
resting cardiac output, not coronary circulation.

4.21   Heart rate   Answers: ACD
There is a resting vague tone on the heart, which is lost after denervation,
and so the heart rate increases. Adenosine induces heart block and if
given in sufficient doses can cause transient asystole. Salbutamol and
adrenaline have β effects causing a tachycardia. Metronidazole has no
effect on the heart rate.

4.22   Answers: DE
Heart rate x stroke volume = cardiac output
Cardiac output x systemic vascular resistance = blood pressure.
Having an adequate blood pressure does not necessarily equate to tissue
perfusion and the blood pressure may be normal but there still may be
tissue hypoxia.

4.23   Infective organisms   Answers: ABF

4.24   Infections on the ITU   **Answers: ABCD**

Malignant disease may cause a generalised reduction in a patient's immunity as well as causing malnutrition. Abdominal surgery may cause basal atelectasis, pre-disposing the patient to pneumonia. A high FiO_2 causes ciliary dysfunction and so increases the risk of respiratory sepsis. Clostridial diarrhoea is commonly caused by protracted antibiotic use.

4.25   Organisms and antibiotics

A	*Staphylococcus aureus*	3.	flucloxacillin
B	*Bacteroides*	2.	metronidazole
C	*Haemophilus influenzae*	5.	amoxycillin
D	enterococci	4.	vancomycin
E	*Klebsiella pneumoniae*	1.	erythromycin

4.26   Drugs and renal failure   **Answers: CE**

Gentamicin doses should be reduced as the GFR falls, more modern dosing regimens use a single dose of gentamicin and then, using trough levels, the next dose frequency is adjusted accordingly. Digoxin accumulates in renal failure as does the metabolite of pethidine, namely norpethidine, which can rise to toxic levels causing convulsions during prolonged use.

4.27   Sepsis   **Answers: ACDE**

For a diagnosis of sepsis the patient must have two or more of the following:
Temperature > 38°C or < 36°C
Heart rate > 90 bpm
Respiratory rate > 20 bpm or $PaCO_2$ < 32 mmHg (4.2 kPa)
White cell count >12 X 10^9/l or < 4.0 X 10^9/l or > 10% immature band forms.

4.28   Septic shock   **Answers: CE**

In septic shock the cardiac output increases and may maintain the blood pressure initially. Systemic vascular resistance is reduced as the patient vasodilates, which causes reduction in venous return and so the central venous pressure is reduced.

4.29 Adult respiratory distress syndrome Answers: ABCE
Renal failure may well be associated with ARDS especially in the presence of multi-organ failure. It does not however generally cause it. Other causes include acid aspiration, traumas, severe pneumonia and massive blood transfusion.

4.30 Adult respiratory distress syndrome Answers: CDE
In ARDS lung compliance is reduced (the lungs are stiff), this being due to thickening of the alveolar membranes. The patient becomes progressively tachypnoeic and fails to maintain an adequate PaO_2 despite high FiO_2. V/Q mismatch refers to ventilation (V) perfusion (Q) disparities.

4.31 Duration of ECG components

A	PR interval	5.	< 0.12 s
B	QRS duration	1.	0.12 s
C	P wave	3.	< 0.1 s
D	QT interval	2.	< 0.3 s
E	cardiac cycle	4.	1.2 s

4.32 Cardiac pressures (mmHg)

A	left ventricle	6.	120/0
B	right ventricle	1.	20/0
C	left atrium	3.	5/10
D	right atrium	4.	0/4
E	pulmonary artery	5.	20/6
F	aorta	2.	120/80

4.33 Complications of acute tubular necrosis Answer: C
Patients with ATN go into renal failure causing uraemia as well as pulmonary oedema, DIC and multi organ dysfunction. Patients may also become hypocalcaemic. They are acidotic and have raised serum potassium.

4.34 Drug overdose Answers: AC
The first three are all causes of renal failure. Rhabdomyolysis causes myoglobulinaemia. Although calculi may cause post-renal failure this is unlikely in this case and both sides must be totally obstructed.

4.35   Established renal failure   **Answer: F**
Fluid in established renal failure should be limited to the previous day's output added to non-sensible losses, namely 500 ml in a non pyrexial patient. Mannitol will have no effect in established renal failure and peritoneal dialysis is inappropriate. The patient should have veno venous haemodiafiltration.

4.36   Inflammatory response   **Answers: CDE**
Cytokines are naturally occurring polypeptides, which are released in the inflammatory response. They include IL1, IL6, IL8 and TNF (tumour necrosis factor).

4.37   Anti-inflammatory agents   **Answers: All false**
All have been used except sulfametopyrazine but none have an established beneficial effect.

4.38   Oliguric patient   **Answers: BCE**
The correct management of a post-surgery patient with a low output is a full assessment including the abdomen to look for deterioration and so a cause for the oliguria. The majority of patients will be under-filled and so will respond to a fluid challenge.

4.39   Respiratory compromise   **Answers: ABE**
Heparin is indicated in the case of a pulmonary embolism. Morphine will help off load a failing heart as well as acting as an anxiolytic and analgesic. Propranolol may cause deterioration in respiratory function especially in an asthmatic patient.

4.40   Tracheostomy   **Answer: C**
Tracheostomy is a formal operation and should be carried out under controlled circumstances under general anaesthetic. However, percutaneous tracheostomy may be performed under local anaesthetic. Both are very useful in enabling adequate toilet of the lungs and also by reducing dead space may aid 'weaning' off ventilation.

4.41   Indications for ventilation   **Answers: AC**
Indications for ventilation include $pCO_2 > 6.5$ kPa or a rising pCO_2 in the face of acidosis pH < 7.25. Hypoxia with a $PaO_2 < 8$ kPa on an FiO_2 of 50% or more is also an indication.

4.42   Pulse oximetry   Answers: ABD
In carbon monoxide poisoning the carbon monoxide binds irreversibly with haemoglobin causing a spuriously high reading. Errors also occur with methaemoglobinaemia. With acute type 1 respiratory failure and patients on intravenous respiratory stimulants, far from being misleading, pulse oximetry is very helpful to monitor a patient's progress.

4.43   Chest X-ray   Answers: ACD
In severe respiratory compromise the patient should be resuscitated before obtaining a chest film.

4.44   100% Oxygen treatment   Answers: ACD
To obtain an inspired oxygen concentration of 100% one must have a closed circuit with a tightly fitting face mask. This can be obtained by continuous positive airway pressure or positive end expiratory pressure ventilation or in the resuscitation room by having a mask with a reservoir.

4.45   Fat embolus   Answers: BD
Fat embolus occurs in the young patient most commonly after closed long bone fractures. The earliest signs are pyrexia and tachycardia. Dyspnoea, restlessness and confusion occur later. Petechiae characteristically occur over the chest and conjunctival folds. Treatment is supportive with correction of hypoxia and maintenance of fluid balance.

4.46   Paralysis of the left hemi-diaphragm   Answers: BDF
The phrenic nerve is predominantly C5 motor and sectioning causes paralysis of the corresponding hemi-diaphragm. This then has paradoxical movement, rising on inspiration.

4.47   Antero-lateral thoracotomy   Answers: BCD

4.48   Inspiration   Answers: ADE
On inspiration the vertical dimension of the chest increases. The ribs do move up and out however rib 1 is largely exempt from this. Serratus anterior is involved (supplied by the long thoracic nerve).

4.49   **Anterior relations of the intra-thoracic**   **Answers: ABE**
       trachea

4.50   **Left hilum of the lung**   **Answers: ABE**
The contents include the pulmonary artery and upper and lower veins, the main bronchus, and the ligament.

4.51   **Pancoast's tumour**   **Answers: CD**
Pancoast's tumour affects the apices of the lungs and causes destruction of the structures found there. Classically, this will cause a disruption of the sympathetic chain and so a Horner's syndrome. They may involve T1 but are unlikely to affect the phrenic nerve as this is very medial. Being apical they do not cause basal atelectasis.

4.52   **Respiration**   **Answers: ABCE**

4.53   **Metabolic and acid-base balance**

A	the greatest stimulus to breathing	4.	hypercarbia
B	pulmonary embolism	5.	hypocarbia
C	type I respiratory failure	2.	hypoxia
D	tented T waves	1.	hyperkalaemia
E	aspirin overdose	3.	acidosis

The increase in $PaCO_2$ is sensed by way of carbonic anhydrase that converts the CO_2 to HCO_3^- and H^+, the latter crosses the blood-brain barrier and so reduces the local pH stimulating respiration. The stimulation however is the $PaCO_2$.

4.54   **Causes of ventilation/perfusion mismatch**   **Answers: ACD**
Ventilation/perfusion mismatch may be demonstrated with a scan which compares the distribution of inhaled radioisotope with intravenous contrast. The main significance of the test is to show areas ventilated but not perfused e.g. in a pulmonary embolus, and areas perfused but not ventilated e.g. atelectasis.

4.55   **Restrictive lung disorder**   **Answers: ABC**
Restrictive lung disorders are associated with reduced compliance, volumes, transfer factor and PaO_2 may well be reduced especially after exercise.

4.56   Obstructive lung disorder   **Answers: BCDE**
An example of obstructive disorder is COAD, which is mainly a problem of getting the air out of the lungs. Transfer factor is reduced due to alveolar destruction and due to dynamic closure of the large bronchi. On expiration there is an increase in total lung capacity.

4.57   Anterior resection   **Answers: BCDE**
The most pronounced effects of the metabolic response to trauma begin to fall 24 hours after the surgery. Catabolism that accompanies trauma increases urea production and excretion. ADH levels rise as part of the endocrine response to stress. Increased serum cortisol leads to sodium and water retention and potassium loss.

4.58   Antidiuretic hormone   **Answers: BD**
Antidiuretic hormone is secreted by the posterior pituitary and acts via cAMP in response to hypovolaemia, high plasma osmolarity and stress.

4.59   Cardiac output   **Answers: ABCE**
Cardiac output is the product of heart rate and stroke volume. The Fick principle is the standard method of measurement whereby cardiac output is equal to oxygen consumption divided by the arteriovenous oxygen content difference.

4.60   Post-operative hypertension   **Answers: AB**
Pain often causes an elevation of systemic arterial pressure which is related to the wound or often the bladder. The volatile anaesthetic agents do not cause hypertension and epidurals most frequently cause post-operative hypotension.

4.61   Heat loss during a laparotomy   **Answers: ABDE**
Theatre temperature is usually maintained at 22°C but may need to be higher for neonatal surgery. Covering exposed surfaces and humidification will minimise heat loss.

4.62   Hypokalaemia   **Answers: EF**
Hyperkalaemia produces peaked T waves and slows conduction time and inhibits the myocardium leading to ventricular standstill. Acidosis causes a shift of potassium from the intracellular to extracellular compartment. The pancreatic juices are rich in potassium and hence fistulae would lead to considerable loss of potassium.

4.63   Arterial plasma bicarbonate   **Answers: CD**
In respiratory acidosis there is an increase in the hydrogen ion concentration and a rise in pCO_2. Metabolic acidosis is defined as reduction in plasma bicarbonate. In respiratory alkalosis renal compensatory mechanisms excrete bicarbonate and sodium ions.

4.64   Major haemorrhage due to trauma   **Answers: ABDE**
Due to activation of peripheral chemoreceptor and baroreceptor activity, the respiratory and vasomotor centres are stimulated. Increased levels of catecholamines and cortisol cause a rise in serum glucose. The resultant respiratory alkalosis causes a rightward shift of the oxygen-haemoglobin dissociation curve.

4.65   Sepsis   **Answers: BCD**
In sepsis, hyperglycaemia may occur due to failing glucose homeostasis in the liver. This hepatic dysfunction may also cause jaundice especially in a patient on ICU who may have cholestasis for a variety of reasons. Gangrene may be a sequel of noradrenaline, however, it is not a complication of sepsis per se. FDPs (fibrinogen degradation products) are an indication of DIC (disseminated intravascular coagulopathy).

4.66   Prokinetic drugs used on ICU   **Answers: ABE**
Cisapride and erythromycin are prokinetic. Sucralfate and Lansoprazole are used in the ICU setting however they are not prokinetic. Anastrazole is an aromatase inhibitor used in breast cancer.

4.67   Lung compliance   **Answers: CDE**
Normal compliance is 60–85 ml/cm H_2O. Usually, compliance is the combination of lung and chest wall compliance and so is affected by splinting from a distended abdomen.

4.68   Gas transfer   **Answers: CDF**
By analysing the amount of carbon monoxide absorbed from alveolar air into arterial blood then the transfer is calculated. Helium gives the volume of the lung, being calculated using a dilution technique (Fick principle).

4.69   Blood gases   Answer: D
Blood gases are taken from the radial of femoral artery or from an arterial line, the brachial is an end artery and so should be avoided. The oxygen content is calculated by knowing the haemoglobin concentration and also the partial pressure of oxygen in arterial blood. Temperature but not heparin affect blood gases; indeed they must be heparinised to avoid coagulation during analysis.

4.70   Complications of arterial lines   Answers: ABCD

4.71   Answers: BCE
Type 1 failure is where the $PaCO_2$ is low and the patient 'blows off' the CO_2, conversely CO_2 accumulates in type 2 failure. Oxygen saturation does not signify tissue delivery. Bicarbonate may be high despite acidosis in a metabolically compensated respiratory acidosis e.g. a patient with type 2 failure who has been given too much oxygen and so has retained CO_2 due to the reduction in their hypoxic drive.

4.72   Flow volume curves
1	upper airway obstruction	B
2	normal	A
3	obstructive disorder	C
4	restrictive disorder	D

4.73   Swan-Ganz catheters   Answers: ADE
Swan-Ganz catheters are balloon tipped catheters which can measure left atrial pressure. The catheter is advanced until the inflated balloon 'wedges' in a branch of the pulmonary artery (pulmonary capillary wedge pressure). It may be inserted in any large central vein. The normal pulmonary artery pressure is 25/10 mmHg. A thermodilution technique is used to measure cardiac output. Systemic vascular resistance can only be calculated from cardiac output and blood pressure.

ANSWERS – CORE MODULE 5: NEOPLASIA, TECHNIQUES AND OUTCOME OF SURGERY

5.1   Chemotherapy   **Answers: AD**
The following tumours are poorly responsive to chemotherapy: pancreatic carcinoma, melanoma, soft tissue sarcoma, colorectal carcinoma, renal carcinoma, thyroid cancer, gastric and cervical cancer.

5.2   Diagnosis of colorectal tumours   Answers: BC
The haemoccult test is based on the interaction between haematin and hydrogen peroxide resulting in the oxidation of the guaiac reagent. It may detect adenomas and carcinomas although in an asymptomatic population over half of the tumours may yield a false-negative reaction. Other agents that cause a positive test include animal haematin and fruit or vegetables with high peroxidase activity. It may soon be superseded my immunological tests which improve sensitivity.

5.3   Malignant melanoma   Answers: BDF
The excision margins used for the treatment of malignant melanoma depend on the depth of invasion. A 1 cm margin is adequate for a Breslow depth < 0.76 mm, 2 cm for 0.76–1.5 mm and 3 cm clearance for lesions > 1.5 mm. There are no chemotherapeutic agents (single agent or combination) at present which can successfully treat metastatic melanoma. Melanoma may spread to lymph nodes and if affected at the time of diagnosis, en bloc dissection of the nodes is performed.

5.4   Audit   Answers: CE
Audit is the essential obligation of all surgeons. There are funds available from the DOH and each hospital should have an audit office with personnel dedicated to the task of audit. Audit should be considered as a loop or more recently spiral. This is where a problem is addressed and a change implemented. The situation should then be reassessed to see if an improvement has been achieved. The process of audit has been shown to improve clinical practice by its very presence.

5.5   Audit   Answers: CE
Audit is defined as 'The systematic, clinical analysis of the quality of medical care, including the procedures used for diagnosis and treatment, the use of resources, and the resulting outcome and quality of life for the patient'. There are three main elements to audit:
i)   Structure: this refers to the available patient resources.
ii)   Process: this is what is done to the patient.
iii) Outcome: the result of clinical intervention.

5.6   UK breast screening programme   Answers: BE

Breast screening in the United Kingdom is provided for women aged between 50 and 64 years. Approximately 77% of women targeted attended for screening (1.16 million in 1995). The initial screen is two views but subsequent ones are single view repeated every three years at present. No physical examination is carried out at the basic screen but should an abnormality be detected, clinical assessment is performed. Women over the age of 64 years may request mammography screening on demand but uptake is poor (only 20,042 women in 1995).

5.7   Fine needle aspiration cytology (FNAC)   Answers: ABD

The accuracy of FNAC is high when the operator is experienced and the cytologist expert. An acellular specimen is classified as C0, and C5 as malignant. FNAC has a specificity and sensitivity of 95%. It is possible to obtain hormone (oestrogen and progesterone) receptor status on FNAC specimens. A 21G needle is used and therefore cytology can be performed without anaesthesia.

5.8   Mastalgia   Answers: ABDF

Breast discomfort is a common complication, being cyclical or non-cyclical. It is most commonly bilateral and may occur at any age. There is usually no physical abnormality other than diffuse nodularity. When symptoms are interfering with the patient's lifestyle then a variety of drugs may be tried. Oil of evening primrose takes a few months to work (rich source of linoleic acid). It is beneficial in 40% of cases. Other drugs include bromocriptine, danazol and tamoxifen (relieve cyclical mastalgia). Tamoxifen is an anti-oestrogen.

5.9   Consent for minors   Answers: AD

The legal age of consent for medical, surgical or dental treatment is sixteen years or over, as determined by Section 8 of the Family Reform Act 1969. In such cases there is no legal requirement to obtain consent from the parent or guardian. When, however, major or hazardous elective surgery is contemplated, it is wise to discuss with the parents unless the patient refuses permission for this.

5.10   Acutely unconscious patient   Answers: ABC

It is essential to involve relatives or carers in the decision making. In an emergency the clinician should not delay taking action when consent cannot be obtained.

5.11 Informed consent   Answers: ABE

Consent must be given freely under no form of any duress. The task of obtaining consent should not be routinely delegated to a junior, especially if the procedure is complicated or specialised. The new regulations will be that the consent must be taken by the surgeon performing the operation.

5.12 Cutaneous malignant melanoma   Answers: ABE

Melanoma incidence has doubled every 10 years and is now 10 per 100,000 per annum in the UK. There is a familial component (atypical mole syndrome), blue eyes, red hair and pale complexion have been demonstrated to increase risk. It is more common on the body and face in men and on the lower limbs in women.

5.13 Radiotherapy   Answers: BCE

Radiotherapy plays a very important role in palliation. Fractionation with radiotherapy given over several weeks is most effective and allows normal tissues to recover.

5.14 Pain in the terminally ill   Answers: CE

Long-term side-effects of drugs that provide adequate pain relief are immaterial when treating the terminally ill. In children and infants who are terminally ill, pain relief is provided by opiates if indicated. Infusion pumps that delivery subcutaneous or intravenous analgesics avoid peaks and troughs in pain control. Portable pumps allow mobile terminally ill patients in pain to avoid prolonged hospital stay.

5.15 Alpha-fetoprotein levels   Answers: BC

Elevation of serum AFP levels occurs commonly in patients with hepatoma and non-seminomatous germ cell tumours but has not been reported in bladder tumours, cervical carcinoma or lymphoma.

5.16 Serum carcinoembryonic antigen (CEA)   Answers: ABE

CEA is a watersoluble glycoprotein of 200 kDa weight. It is elevated in fewer than 5% of patients with Dukes' grade A colorectal cancer, 25% of Dukes' B and 44% of Dukes' C and approximately 65% of patients with distant metastases. It is not a useful diagnostic marker as it is increased in severe benign liver disease, inflammatory conditions particularly of the gastro-intestinal tract, trauma, infection, collagen diseases, renal impairment and smoking. It can assist in detecting recurrence. The half-life is ten days.

5.17 Basal cell carcinoma   Answers: AB

Basal cell carcinoma is the most common skin tumour, occurring more frequently in men. It is usually single but can be multiple and may be inherited in an autosomal dominant fashion. Classically, it is a nodular lesion. A 0.5 cm margin is usually sufficient. Radiotherapy has been used but should be avoided near cartilage.

5.18 Breast carcinoma   Answers: ABDEFGH

Various pathological measurements influence prognosis. Nodal status is the single most important factor. Grade, size, lymphovascular invasion, EGF receptor, oestrogen receptor all have prognostic influence. In situ carcinoma is associated with local recurrence but not poor survival.

5.19 Gastric cancer   Answer: C

Gastric cancer is clearly linked to low socio-economic class, is twice as common in men as in women and is more common in individuals with blood group A. Its highest incidence is in Japan where routine screening with gastroscopy is employed and gastric surgery is at its most refined. Consequently, mortality rates are reduced.

5.20 Oesophageal cancer   Answers: ABCF

Most oesophageal cancers are squamous carcinomas. A number of factors are important in the aetiology including dietary factors, particularly high nitrosamine intake, vitamin A and C deficiencies, certain trace element deficiencies and the consumption of mouldy food contaminated by aflatoxins. Other proven associations include smoking and alcohol consumption, factors causing stasis such as webs and achalasia, and Barrett's metaplasia. FAP is associated with colorectal carcinoma and also gastric, duodenal and pancreatic carcinoma.

5.21 Tumours and serum markers **Answers: AD**

The tumour marker for ovarian cancer is CA125. Medullary thyroid cancer arises from C-cells and therefore calcitonin is a useful marker for the disease. Alpha-fetoprotein is synthesised by embryonal hepatocytes and elevated in 80% of patients with hepatocellular carcinoma. Alpha-fetoprotein and hCG are tumour markers for testicular cancer.

These tumour markers are non-specific. They are useful in staging the disease and detecting recurrence.

5.22 Colorectal cancer **Answers: All false**

Familial polyposis coli is an autosomal dominant disorder. Affected individuals have multiple large bowel polyps with a tendency to malignant transformation which becomes inevitable over approximately 20 years. Previously the average life expectancy has been 42 years. Colonoscopic screening of family members from the age of 16 and prophylactic colectomy or panproctocolectomy for affected individuals are changing this. In the UK, colorectal cancer is now second only to lung cancer as a cause of death from malignant disease. It accounts for 95% of large bowel cancers, the remainder being anal tumours. Although p53 gene mutations are the most commonly seen genetic defect in colorectal cancer, development of cancer is a multi-step process and requires more than one genetic change.

5.23 *Helicobacter pylori* **Answers: BCEF**

Helicobacter pylori is found in up to 50% of stomachs world-wide. Its attack on gastric mucosa is responsible for the susceptibility of infected individuals to peptic ulceration and it is found superficially within the mucosa. It can be thus identified in gastric biopsies and also detected serologically and by a variety of enzyme mediated assays exploiting the organism's secretion of urease. A variety of eradication regimes exist of which the most cost effective is with omeprazole, amoxycillin and metronidazole.

5.24 Malignant melanoma   Answer: A

The vast majority of malignant melanomas arise in previously normal skin. The Breslow thickness, of the melanoma in mm, has been demonstrated to better predict prognosis than Clark's levels which refer less precisely to the histological level to which the tumour has penetrated the skin. Lesions greater than 1 mm thick need only a 3 cm excision margin, no improvement in either survival or local recurrence rates have been found for more radical surgery. Lentigo maligna is a pigmented lesion with invasive potential arising in sun-damaged skin, mainly in the elderly. Malignant change in such lesions takes between 10 and 30 years to develop.

5.25 Carcinogens and malignancies   Answers: ACE

Aromatic amines such as β naphthylamine are associated with urinary tract, especially bladder tumours, in chemical workers particularly involved with dyes and pesticides. Benzene exposure of painters, printers, mechanics and others working with petroleum derivatives and organic solvents is associated with leukaemias and lymphatic cancers. Arsenic is used in pesticide manufacture and exposure also occurs in metal smelters, it is associated with skin and lung cancers as well as bladder tumours.

5.26 Cancer registries   Answers: ADE

Cancer registries obtain their data by identifying all death certificates which state cancer as the cause of or contributing to death and studying the notes of these patients. Post-mortem findings contribute greatly to the accuracy of such data. Amongst other things cancer registries can monitor the outcomes of ongoing treatment trials and compare current therapies and centres. In addition, they enable at-risk families to be identified for study and possibly screening. Whilst they are a source of valuable local data they are of particular value as a source of large numbers with national data for study enabling national features and trends to be identified and studied and regional variations to be highlighted.

5.27   Hamartomas   **Answers: ACD**

Hamartomas are benign masses made up of fully differentiated normal components of the tissues in which they arise. In a hamartoma the proportion and composition of these normal tissue components differs greatly from the normal tissue structure. The most common hamartomas are vascular and include birth marks such as port wine stains. The polyps of Peutz-Jeghers syndrome are gastrointestinal hamartomas, whilst the associated lesion at the vermilion border of the lips is increased pigmentation. Although not neoplastic they are mass lesions, the presentation of Peutz-Jeghers syndrome is often with intussusception or intestinal obstruction caused by the mass lesions. Unlike true neoplasms they cannot grow autonomously.

5.28   Adenomas   **Answer: A**

Adenomas are benign tumours of ductal or glandular epithelial cells. Consistent with their benign nature they are typically encapsulated and not invasive. Invasion and cellular nuclear pleomorphism are characteristics of malignancy. Annular lesions which grow around hollow organs and can cause stricturing are typically malignant. Neoplasms of squamous, columnar or transitional epithelial cells are papillomata if benign or carcinomas if malignant. However, it is thought that there are no truly benign transitional cell papillomas.

5.29   A $T_2N_1M_0$ tumour   **Answer: B** ⟱ .

A Dukes' B colorectal cancer has invaded through the bowel wall but does not involve lymph nodes, (N_0). N_1 stage breast cancer indicates ipsilateral mobile axillary lymphadenopathy. Typically the extent of loco-regional nodal disease is a more important indicator of prognosis than tumour size, hence a T_2N_1 tumour will generally have a better prognosis than a T_1N_2 tumour. Evidence of regional node involvement is an indicator for radiotherapy or chemotherapy in many cancers.

5.30 Dukes' staging of colorectal cancer   Answers: BDE

Dukes' classification is based on histological findings and hence is unknown prior to surgery. Dukes' classification has no stage D. However, stage D is a commonly used term for metastatic disease. One must remember that even patients with a Dukes' A tumour may die as a result of metastases in later years and 5% are dead within five years.

DUKES' STAGE	TUMOUR	NODES	5 YEAR SURVIVAL
A	Confined to bowel wall	Negative	90%
B	Breaching muscularis propria	Negative	70%
C1		Positive	40%
C2		Apical node positive	25%

5.31 Bronchial carcinoma   Answers: ABC

Bronchial carcinoma is currently the most common cause of death from malignancy in the UK. Clinical features include a persistent cough, haemoptysis, atypical or recurrent chest infections and weight loss. Hoarseness generally results from involvement of the recurrent laryngeal nerve and ptosis is a feature of Horner's syndrome indicating involvement of the cervical sympathetic plexus by an apical or Pancoast tumour. Sister Joseph's nodule is a malignant nodule arising at the umbilicus from an abdominal malignancy such as gastric, colonic or ovarian cancer but cutaneous metastases from lung cancer can occur anywhere. Bronchial carcinoma is associated with hypertrophic pulmonary osteodystrophy. Sudeck's atrophy is the end stage of post-traumatic algodystrophy.

5.32   Rectal carcinoma   Answers: BDE

Left-sided colonic lesions are more likely to present with obstruction because of a generally narrower lumen and more solid bowel content. Anaemia is a feature of a right-sided lesion where chronic blood loss may go unnoticed without faecal occult blood tests and where particularly caecal lesions can reach quite a size without causing obstruction. Fresh or altered rectal bleeding is generally apparent with a rectal carcinoma. Melaena is a feature of an upper GI bleed where at least a moderate quantity of blood has been lost and altered by digestion and passage through the gut. Tenesmus is painful, ineffective calls to stool.

5.33   Management of malignant disease   Answers: BCF

Staging for Hodgkin's disease is by CT or laparoscopy. Extensive surgery for inoperable disease is not justified because the expected survival may be limited but may be justified when there is the imminent risk of intestinal obstruction.

5.34   CT scanning in malignant disease   Answers: CE

CT can only reliably demonstrate metastases in the liver once they are over 2 cm. Recurrent disease may appear as surgical scarring and appearances do not necessarily correspond to surgical resectability.

5.35   Oncogenes   Answers: ABE

Oncogenes are normal cellular genes with the potential to cause malignant transformation when structurally and functionally mutated or abnormally or inappropriately expressed. They tend to have gene products involved in key cellular regulatory processes. They can cause malignancy, not only when the gene product is altered by mutation, but when they are over or under-expressed or expressed at an inappropriate stage of the cell cycle. Because of the key regulatory roles of their products they tend to be fundamental to cellular activity and hence highly conserved throughout evolution. Their discovery and much research work hinged on the discovery of tumour viruses containing viral analogues of these genes, derived from cellular oncogenes, and acting as vectors for their transmission to and malignant transformation of host cells. The H-ras oncogene in the Harvey murine sarcoma virus is found in a variety of common human cancers.

5.36   Tumour suppressor genes   **Answers: ADEF**

The most well known tumour suppressor genes include p53 and the retinoblastoma genes. Mutations of the p53 gene are the most common genetic change seen in colorectal cancers. Tumour suppressor gene products normally regulate excessive cellular proliferation. Therefore loss of function of both genes is required before cell proliferation is deregulated and hence tumour suppressor gene mutations act in a recessive manner to produce neoplastic transformation. p53 protein binds a specific DNA sequence which activates transcription of adjacent genes whose products inhibit cell proliferation. Some other tumour suppressor genes are in this class encoding DNA-binding transcription activating proteins. p53 also functions to prevent transmission of mutations by several mechanisms including facilitating apoptosis, programmed cell death, preventing replication of cells whose DNA has been damaged but not repaired.

5.37   Neoplastic cells   **Answers: ABC**

To establish and proliferate in a new site tumour cells must ensure an adequate blood supply. Metastasis is facilitated by the ability of neoplastic cells to secrete angiogenic and angioproliferative factors to promote development of new blood vessels and hence their own blood supply. To metastasise cells must overcome their normal cohesion and be able to invade the tissue, a property facilitated by the secretion of the enzyme protease. Cancer cells must adhere to the basement membrane in order to pass through, and invade from the epithelium. Adhesion to the basement membrane requires the expression of integrins, cell surface receptors for basement membrane components, but not cadherins which enhance cell to cell adhesion.

5.38   Cell cycle   **Answer: D**

In the cell cycle the growth and proliferation of normal cells is regulated and changes in the regulatory mechanisms may result in neoplastic transformation. Immediately following cell division cells enter the G_1 phase of high metabolic activity but no DNA synthesis. DNA is synthesised in the next stage, the S stage. From there the cell enters the G_2 stage preparing for the M stage, or mitosis, which as the DNA content of the cell is now double results in the production of two diploid cells. All the stages apart from G_1 have fairly fixed durations and hence the growth rate of tissue depends on the length of time its cells spend in this stage.

5.39   Features of malignancy   Answers: CDE

Features of malignancy at a cellular level include nuclear hyper-chromasia, a high nuclear to cytoplasmic ratio, nuclear pleomorphism, an increased mitotic rate and an increased incidence of abnormal mitoses. Such changes throughout the width of an epithelium would constitute carcinoma in situ, only when invasion occurs and the cells traverse the basement membrane as malignancy developed.

5.40   Screening test   Answer: E

The specificity of a screening test depends on its ability to correctly identify those tested who do not have the condition in question. Thus a highly specific test would have a low false positive rate and a high true negative rate. The number of true positives is a measure of the sensitivity of the test. A valuable test would have a high specificity and high sensitivity. PSA is elevated in at least half of all cases of benign prostatic hypertrophy and thus of no value in population screening for prostatic cancer due to the high rate of false positives that would result. Screening is appropriate where early detection will significantly improve outcome and modify treatment requirements and associated morbidity or influence reproductive choices. Colonoscopy will detect early and pre-malignant colorectal lesions with a high sensitivity and specificity. However, because of the cost, preparation and poor acceptability to patients it is only appropriate for screening high risk groups.

5.41   Chemotherapy toxicity   Answers: BCD

Combination chemotherapy is utilised to combat drug resistance, combinations of drugs are selected to have the minimum of overlapping toxicities but its use is at least as toxic if not more so than a single agent. Many agents, particularly doxorubicin and Vinca alkaloids are predominantly metabolised in the liver. When liver function is impaired excretion is reduced and unless doses are adjusted toxicity will be increased. Highly emetogenic drugs require treatment often by infusion with the 5HT or serotonin antagonists, of which ondansetron is the most common example. Bone marrow suppression may be indicated by bleeding such as epistaxis due to thrombocytopenia/pancytopenia. Hair loss due to chemotherapy is always reversible after treatment even if the quality of re-growth may be altered.

5.42   Tumour markers   **Answers: ACDE**
Tumour markers may have various roles in different tumours including diagnosis, monitoring and staging. aFP and bhCG are useful in both detecting and monitoring ovarian germ cell tumours. CEA is not sufficiently specific or sensitive to be useful in screening for colorectal cancer but it is valuable in monitoring recurrence. Its serum level is only raised in 5% of Dukes' A cases, rising to 65% of those with metastic colorectal carcinomas. The same is true of the role of PSA in prostatic carcinoma and CA125 in ovarian carcinoma. Serum FP levels are raised in up to 80% of patients with hepatocellular carcinoma. Its measurement is thus of value in screening high risk groups such as those with hepatitis B and cirrhosis patients and high risk populations such as the Chinese.

5.43   Treatment of malignancies   **Answers: ACDEF**
Octreotide is an analogue of somatostatin used to relieve symptoms associated with carcinoid tumours, VIPomas and glucagonomas. Goserelin is an analogue of gonadorelin used to suppress gonadal hormone secretion in the management of prostatic and breast cancers. Cyproterone is also used in the treatment of prostatic cancer but because of its action of competitive inhibition of testosterone, it is however a progesterone analogue. Aminoglutethimide inhibits conversion of cholesterol to pregnenolone reducing all steroid hormone production and inhibits conversion of androgens to oestrogens in peripheral tissues and is used in the treatment of breast cancer. Megestrol is a progesterone analogue used in the second and third-line treatment of breast and endometrial cancers.

5.44   Radiotherapy   Answer: CE

Radiotherapy and chemotherapy are the treatment for anal squamous cell carcinoma. Surgery is reserved for salvage procedures or tiny and premalignant lesions. In Dukes' C rectal cancers radiotherapy reduces the local recurrence rate but does not improve survival. Oral cancers have frequently spread to cervical lymph nodes at presentation and the sensitivity of the disease to radiotherapy can enable regional control to be achieved whilst avoiding disfiguring surgery. Radiotherapy causes oxygen-dependent tissue damage. Fractionation enables smaller doses to be given at each session such that slow growing tissues (e.g. nerves) have more chance between fractions to repair the reduced amount of damage so caused and enables rapidly proliferation tissues to recover, more rapidly than tumour between fractions. In addition to the reduced amount of normal tissue damage, fractionation ensures that tumour bulk is reduced with each dose. Areas that were originally hypoxic become oxygenated and more readily destroyed by radiotherapy, thus improving tumour response rates.

5.45   Early complications of radiotherapy   Answers: ACEG

The early complications of radiotherapy reflect the sensitivity of rapidly growing cells to radiation damage. They include desquamation lesions of the skin and gastrointestinal tract (inflammation, bleeding and ulceration) infertility and bone marrow suppression. Hypothyroidism is a late complication of exposure of the thyroid gland to radiation and may also complicate radio-iodine treatment for thyroid malignancy. The production of secondary malignancies is now recognised as a late complication of radiotherapy and may be seen to develop from three years post therapy. Acute leukaemias are the most common although the incidence of solid tumours is also increased in individuals treated with radiotherapy.

5.46   Hypercalcaemia   Answers: ABDEF

Hypercalcaemia is most commonly caused by hyperparathyroidism and malignancy. It usually occurs in malignancy with bony metastases, a feature of some of the most common tumours. A positive Chvostek's sign is a feature of hypocalcaemia. Features of hypercalcaemia include bone pain, renal stones, malaise and depression (moans) and abdominal pain (groans) and peptic ulceration.

5.47   The breast   Answer: C

The breast lies between the 2nd and the 6th ribs, overlying the pectoralis major, external oblique and serratus anterior muscles. Between the breast and pectoralis major is the submammary space. This is formed between a condensed layer of superficial fascia (a continuation of Scarpa's fascia on which the breast directly lies) and the deep fascia overlying the muscle. The breast receives its blood supply from branches of the internal thoracic, lateral thoracic and intercostal arteries as well as pectoral branches of the thoracoacromial artery. Most of the lymphatic drainage from the lateral half of the breast is to the axillary and infraclavicular nodes but lymph may also flow to the medial half of the breast and internal thoracic nodes as well as to the opposite breast, cervical nodes and peritoneal cavity. The latter becoming increasingly used when the more usual pathways are obstructed.

5.48   Gynaecomastia   Answers: BE

Bromocriptine inhibits prolactin secretion and is used to suppress lactation and in the treatment of galactorrhoea. Cimetidine is an H$_2$-antagonist used in dyspepsia, it also interferes with liver metabolism and may cause raised oestrogen levels sufficient to promote gynaecomastia particularly in the elderly and at high dosage. Similarly liver disease including cirrhosis can cause oestrogen/androgen imbalance and gynaecomastia. Oral corticosteroids may cause Cushing's syndrome but not gynaecomastia. Parathyroid gland tumours affect calcium metabolism, pituitary tumours and hyperthyroidism may cause gynaecomastia.

5.49   Breast abscess   Answers: BD

Incision and drainage is the treatment for breast abscesses. However, early use of antibiotics may prevent a breast abscess developing to this stage and antibiotics help to speed up resolution following drainage. Commonly used antibiotics include flucloxacillin, penicillin, metronidazole and Augmentin. Tetracycline is rarely indicated in pregnancy and breast feeding. Small abscesses may be managed with aspiration, which may need repeating and antibiotics. Breast feeding need not be discontinued unless it is too painful, in which case milk should be expressed (if this is easier) or lactation suppressed. Neither appropriate antibiotics or bacteria in the milk have been shown to harm the baby. Smoking alters breast tissue circulation and oxygenation and is associated with periductal mastitis, complication of which causes most fistula formation. Although special precautions may be needed depending upon the stage of pregnancy and CNS depressants should be used with caution, pregnancy is not a contraindication to general anaesthesia.

5.50   Mammography   Answers: CDE

Mammography has a false negative rate of 15%. Negative cytology or histology and a consistent clinical picture are thus required to determine correct management of a breast lump. Where there is doubt on mammography, ultrasonography is used for its superior ability to differentiate cystic from solid lesions. Analysis of results from the first few years of the National Breast Screening Programme demonstrated that significantly more cancers were detected if two views were taken and this is what all women now entering the Programme have at the first visit. The risk of a single view mammogram inducing a fatal breast cancer is estimated to be around 1 in 105. The NBSP is currently restricted to women between 50 and 64 years of age.

5.51   Fibroadenoma   Answers: CE

Fibroadenoma do not undergo cyclical change. They occur most commonly in women aged 18-25, although they are responsible for 15% of palpable lumps in 30-40 year olds. They may be multiple and are mobile. Many spontaneously regress.

5.52   Breast pain   Answers: ADE

Pre-menstrual breast pain is common and does not signify that there is sinister disease present. Pain occurs in about 1 in 10 operable breast cancers and more frequently in advanced disease. Pain is most commonly cyclical. Teitze's syndrome, or costochondritis, is a cause of non-cyclical breast pain. Severe cyclical breast pain may respond to hormonal manipulation with tamoxifen, bromocriptine and danazol.

5.53   Fine needle aspiration cytology   Answer: A

All patients presenting with a breast lump should undergo an FNA if excision biopsy is not indicated, in addition to clinical assessment and mammography or ultrasonography. Ideally it should be performed after mammography as it can cause distortion and interfere with the interpretation. Malignant, cellularly dense lesions are much more likely to yield a positive FNA than benign lesions. Consequently an acellular aspirate from a clinically and radiologically benign lesion in a young woman may not warrant repeating. Cystic fluid need only be sent for histology if it is bloody, routine cytology is generally unhelpful.

5.54   Fibroadenoma   Answer: B

Fibroadenoma are not true neoplasms as they do not develop from a single breast cell but from a single lobule. They occur most commonly in women in their 20s when cancer is rare but as they may be misdiagnosed in up to half of cases an FNA should be performed. Mammography is not generally appropriate in women under 35. Provided examination, FNA and mammography are satisfactory it is acceptable to observe these lesions in older women not wanting excision. Carcinoma rarely develops in fibroadenoma, the incidence is approximately 1 in 103. When bigger than 5 cm they are known as giant fibroadenoma. Phylloides tumours are fibroadenoma-like lesions and, histologically, are more commonly benign but can be malignant and can become extremely large.

5.55   Breast cancer   Answers: ACEG

Atypical ductal hyperplasia is the one benign breast condition with a significant risk of subsequent malignancy. Sufferers have a 4–5 times increased risk of developing cancer, a risk further increased if they also have a positive family history. The incidence of breast cancer is increased in women with an early menarche and late menopause, nullipars and those having their first child over the age of 35. Obesity is also associated with a significantly increased risk probably because of increased conversion of androgens to oestrogens in this tissue and an increased risk with diets high in saturated fats. Oophorectomy reduces oestrogen exposure and is used as adjuvant therapy for breast cancer in premenopausal women.

5.56   Nipple discharge   Answer: A

Nipple discharge, even in non-lactating women, is a physiological occurrence but pathological causes of discharge include duct ectasia and periductal mastitis, duct papilloma, carcinoma and galactorrhoea. Both papillomas and carcinomas commonly cause a blood-stained discharge. A total duct excision is only required for persistent, problematic discharge from multiple ducts, dependent upon the cause, antibiotics or microductectomy may be appropriate treatments.

5.57   Axilla   Answers: BCD

The axillary tail of the breast lies on the medial axillary wall. Within the axilla there are an average of 35 lymph nodes, although there may be over 50 in a level three axillary clearance. The axillary vein lies medial to the artery and the brachial plexus and is a useful surgical landmark to avoiding these structures, particularly in axillary sampling. Pectoralis minor divides the axillary nodes into three levels, below, behind and above the muscle. The muscle need only be retracted for axillary sampling when level I and II nodes are removed but is excised for a level III axillary clearance. Division of the intercostobrachial nerve (T1) causes anaesthesia of the skin of the floor of the axilla and medial aspect of the upper arm.

5.58   Wide local excision and axillary dissection   Answers: BCD

Wide local excision, axillary dissection and post-operative radiotherapy are less mutilating than mastectomy. Some women who have breast conservation procedures have psychological fears concerning recurrence. Radiotherapy to the breast is required post-operatively to ensure acceptable rates of local disease control. It is necessary to check that the histology of a wide local excision specimen includes resection margins of at least 2 cm and many operators confirm microscopic tumour clearance by taking cavity wall biopsies. The advantage of axillary dissection over radiotherapy is that it offers accurate staging, and the most important prognostic factor for breast cancer and the feature most likely to dictate the use of chemotherapy is axillary lymph node status. Ductal carcinoma in-situ is often associated with invasive carcinoma, and although it is a premalignant condition when treated with local excision around a third of patients developed subsequent invasive carcinoma in the residual breast tissue. It is therefore best treated with subcutaneous or simple mastectomy.

5.59   Malignancy on mammograms   Answers: ACD

Features of malignancy on mammography include spiculation, tentaculation, fine scattered microcalcification (looking like salt sprinkled on film), skin thickening and some distortion of normal breast architecture. Although diagnostic accuracy may be improved by taking two views and combining the test with ultrasonography all of these features may occur in some benign lesions and a diagnosis must always be confirmed by FNA or excision biopsy. Well defined smooth margins suggestive of encapsulation suggest that the lesion is benign.

5.60   Tamoxifen   Answers: CDEF

Tamoxifen is an oestrogen receptor antagonist. There is no benefit if treatment is continued for more than five years. Although treatment for at least two years produces better results than shorter courses and some studies using tamoxifen for more than two years at more than 20 mg/day have shown an increase in the incidence of endometrial cancer in such patients, it has yet to be established whether acceptable outcomes can be achieved with treatment for more than two but less than five years. Treatment is thus currently recommended for five years. In elderly patients unfit or unwilling to undergo surgery, tamoxifen may cause regression of the tumour or at least halt progression sufficiently to allow the patient to be symptom free and die from other causes.

5.61 Male breast cancer — Answers: BE

Male breast cancer accounts for less than 1% of all breast cancer cases. Stage for stage its prognosis is the same as in women though male breast cancer tends to present at a more advanced stage. There is no association between gynaecomastia and breast cancer. However, there is an increased incidence in males with Klinefelter's syndrome with the chromosomal abnormality 46XXY. Despite the different male hormonal environment the cancer responds to tamoxifen and although the usual treatment is a radical mastectomy advanced disease may respond well to orchidectomy.

5.62 Palpable breast cysts — Answers: AB

Typically breast cysts are smooth and fluctuant but they may mimic cancer by being non-fluctuant and causing skin tethering. At least half the patients with breast cysts will have two or more, commonly bilaterally. They are most common in women in their 40s (their fifth decade). A cyst which has refilled following initial aspiration may be re-aspirated at follow-up but one which refills more than twice should be excised because it indicates an increased risk of an underlying carcinoma.

5.63 Paget's disease of the breast — Answers: BE

Paget's disease is infiltration of the nipple skin by distinctive large clear carcinoma cells associated with an underlying invasive or intraductal carcinoma. In its early stages the scaly erythematous skin changes around the nipple may be mistaken for eczema. Because of its infiltrative nature and malignant progression the best survival and local recurrence rates are achieved with mastectomy and axillary clearance. Secondary sarcoma development is a feature of Paget's disease of bone.

5.64 Routine investigations for a patient with breast cancer — Answer: A

A routine chest X-ray in all patients diagnosed with breast cancer is useful to detect pulmonary metastases. Other scans should not be used routinely as detection rates are low. Only with T3 and T4 tumours are metastases sufficiently likely to justify routine bone scans and liver ultrasound scans, especially as their detection may modify proposed treatment. CT scans are only used when clinically indicated. Tumour markers are not routinely used in staging breast cancer.

5.65   Breast cancer   Answers: All false
Despite features such as skin tethering, fixation, nipple retraction and axillary lymphadenopathy being more usual features of malignant than benign breast disease they are not pathognomonic of malignancy and may occur in other infective and benign breast conditions. Further, mammography may be falsely suggestive of malignancy in around 1% of cases and even when two view mammography, ultrasonography and FNA are employed it may still be necessary on occasion to perform excision biopsy to make a certain diagnosis. Such diagnostic uncertainty emphasises the need to obtain a histological diagnosis before undertaking surgery for breast cancer.

5.66   Managing screen detected breast legions   Answers: BCE
Screen detected lesions are small, early tumours and often difficult to assess histologically. It is important that the best possible assessment is facilitated. Frozen sectioning may cause distortion and make a precise diagnosis impossible, therefore formalin fixation and paraffin embedding prior to sectioning of the specimen must always be used in these cases. Surgical excision of these lesions can be guided either by insertion of a needle and positioning of a guide-wire or injection of a mixture of radio-opaque and coloured dyes into the lesion under mammographic control. Due to a degree of diffusion of the dye within breast tissue the guide-wire technique is more accurate, although with an experienced operator results can be equally good with both methods. It is important to ensure excision by sending the specimen for radiographic confirmation that the abnormality is within the specimen before the operation is completed. It is essential to have a histological diagnosis on a radiologically suspicious lesion. This may be obtained by stereotactic core biopsy.

5.67   Breast reconstruction   Answers: ABD
A prosthesis, if it is to be used, should be inserted beneath pectoralis major to reduce poor cosmetic results from capsule contraction, and creating a pocket inferiorly to ensure that it lies and remains at the appropriate level. Reconstructive techniques may be useful in salvage surgery where a large amount of tissue may need to be removed leaving a large defect. Radiotherapy does not cause significant damage to the large pedicle blood vessels of a flap and may be included in a field of radiation which may be of particular relevance when used for salvage procedures.

5.68   Adjuvant therapy for breast cancer   Answers: ACDEF

Prognosis in breast cancer patients depends on the presence of micrometastases at the time of surgery. Tamoxifen, when used as first line adjuvant therapy in early breast cancer, reduces both recurrence and death rates and although the effect is greatest in postmenopausal women and oestrogen receptor positive tumours, it is also of significant benefit in premenopausal women and oestrogen receptor negative tumours. In premenopausal women the annual mortality and recurrence rates can both be reduced by a quarter by having ovarian ablation (either by surgery, radiation or chemical suppression). Slightly higher reductions of annual mortality and recurrence rates have been demonstrated with the use of combination chemotherapy, with the greatest benefits being found in premenopausal women. CMF, cyclophosphamide, methotrexate and 5-fluoro-uracil, is the combination of chemotherapeutic agents most commonly used. Finasteride is used in benign prostatic hyperplasia. Cyproterone is used in the treatment of prostatic cancer.

**5.69   The UICC TNM classification of breast   Answers: ACE
          cancer**

TNM classification for breast cancer

Stage	Tumour size	Stage	Node involvement
T_1	up to 2cm	N_1	Ipsilateral mobile axillary nodes
T_2	> 2 cm but < 5 cm	N_2	Ipsilateral fixed axillary nodes
T_3	> 5 cm	N_3	Ipsilateral internal mammary nodes
T_4	Any size with chest wall or skin involvement		

Comparison of TNM and Manchester classification

TNM	Manchester
$T_0 - T_1$	Stage I
$N_0 - N_1$	
T_2, N_1	Stage II
$T_3 - T_4$	Stage III
$N_2 - N_3$	
M_1	Stage IV

The UICC is the International Union Against Cancer.

5.70   Metastatic breast carcinoma   Answers: ABCDE
Vomiting is a common side-effect of opiates likely to be required for analgesia in this situation. Breast cancer commonly metastasises to bone and malignant hypercalcaemia is thus common. The brain is also a common site for breast cancer metastases where tumour volume and associated peri-tumour oedema cause raised intracranial pressure. Extensive liver metastases can compress the stomach impairing emptying and causing vomiting. Constipation may particularly be associated with opiate analgesics although intra-abdominal disease and ascites may contribute; it may then cause obstructive symptoms including vomiting.

5.71   Pain relief in terminally ill cancer patients   Answers: DE
It is helpful to patients to be realistic about what can be achieved in pain management and whilst most pain can be controlled and all terminally ill patients should be pain free at night it may not be possible to relieve pain in someone terminally ill when they are active. The relief of pain may involve the use of radiotherapy, antidepressants, anticonvulsants, anaesthetic techniques, steroids and a range of alternative therapies in addition to analgesics. Analgesia when used is best given regularly as terminal pain tends to be constant in nature and it avoids distressing breakthrough of pain, control of which may be harder to regain. Subcutaneous infusion is a useful route in terminal care and can easily be managed outside of a hospital situation. Although there is fear of causing respiratory suppression with opiates, they reduce respiratory demand and hence decrease breathlessness as well as helping to reduce secretions and suppress coughs.

5.72   Common side-effects of opiates   Answers: ABDE
Opiates have selective depressant and excitatory actions on various CNS centres. The most common shared side-effects of opiates are constipation, nausea, vomiting and drowsiness. Other adverse effects include dry mouth, sweating, hypotension, headache and physical dependence.

5.73   Terminal care bone pain   Answers: AB
In terminal care radiotherapy can be useful not only for managing bone pain but for reducing symptoms related to tumour bulk in surgically inaccessible or hazardous areas and reducing inoperable fungating lesions. Whilst steroids such as dexamethasone are useful in reducing problems due to peri-tumour oedema, especially where cerebral and spinal metastases are concerned, steroids are not useful for bone pain per se and steroid usage may be complicated by osteoporosis, and even pathological fracture, exacerbating bone and joint pain. Steroid injections, often combined with local anaesthetic, may be useful when given into joints and specific pain trigger spots. Although recognition and treatment of a patient's depression may improve their tolerance of pain, antidepressants are not a specific treatment for bone pain. The antidepressant amitriptyline is useful in the treatment of neuralgia. Transcutaneous Electrical Nerve Stimulation may help in the management of pain due to nerve compression or destruction.

5.74   Breast reconstruction   Answers: ADE
A latissimus dorsi flap can be used following a subcutaneous mastectomy if a de-epithelialised flap is used. It is commonly used in conjunction with a prosthesis to add bulk and shape to the breast. The thoracodorsal nerve is often transected to prevent contracture of the muscle. The second intercostobrachial nerve is often sacrificed and the patient must be informed pre-operatively of the ensuing numbness.

5.75   Palpable breast lump   Answer: E
Breast lumps in this age may be cysts or carcinoma. Triple assessment should be performed (clinical examination, FNAC and mammography/ ultrasound). Mammography alone has a sensitivity of 86%, clinical examination alone 86% and FNAC 95%. However, in combination there is a positive predictive value of 98%. DCIS is impalpable and is seen on mammography or specimens only. 10% breast cancer has a genetic predisposition – autosomal dominant with incomplete penetrance, therefore transmission is by either sex.

5.76 Drugs ideal for continuous subcutaneous infusion

Answers: BC

Diamorphine is preferable to morphine by this route because of its increased solubility and hence lower delivery volume. Whilst amitriptyline and domperidone are effective for these respective problems they are not suitable for subcutaneous infusion. Haloperidol or cyclizine would be suitable anti-emetics.

5.77 Post-operative confusion

Answers: ABCDEF

Post-operative confusion is common, especially in elderly patients. Causes include disorientation with a strange environment, cerebral and peripheral organ ischaemia secondary to hypotension or anaemia, drugs such as benzodiazepines and opiates, alcohol withdrawal, electrolyte disturbances and sepsis especially where the release of toxins from necrotic material is involved.

5.78 Informed consent

Answers: BC

Not only common or rare but extremely serious complications must be discussed with the patient. Although a colostomy is a serious undertaking for a patient it is so unlikely to be required for a right hemi-colectomy that its discussion is more likely to cause unnecessary anxiety. The same would not be true of a left hemi-colectomy or anterior resection. The incidence of post-ERCP pancreatitis is between 1 and 3% and is a potentially fatal condition. Whilst it may seem apparent that a patient, by submitting, has consented to a procedure under local anaesthetic, a consent form provides some evidence that an attempt was made to both explain the procedure and ensure that the patient understood the procedure adequately for informed consent. However, a consent form is only evidence that some attempt was made to obtain informed consent, not that this was correctly obtained. It is not necessary to give the same information to all patients but what is appropriate to their understanding, individual risks, professional and personal circumstances.

5.79   Gynaecomastia   **Answers: CD**

Gynaecomastia is the most common condition affecting the male breast and is the enlargement of the ductal and stromal tissues. It is benign and usually reversible. Malignancy should be suspected if the area is hard, eccentric or ulcerated. Most patients have a hormone imbalance. Treatment involves discontinuing drugs causing gynaecomastia. Tamoxifen and danazol have been tried with variable results. Surgical removal is indicated for failure of medical treatment or cosmesis.

5.80   Patient with nipple discharge   **Answers: BD**

Bloody nipple discharge is serious and one should always attempt to exclude an underlying carcinoma. Blood stained discharge is most frequently due to epithelial hyperplasia in the form of a duct papilloma. Duct ectasia also causes bloody discharge but is less common. Hyperprolactinaemia causes galactorrhoea. Investigation should include Haemostix testing for blood, cytological examination and assessment of the breast with examination and mammography. Microdochectomy is used for single discharging duct and total duct excision for multiple duct discharge. Total duct excision is Hadfield's operation.

5.81   Unconscious patient following road   **Answers: ACD**
**   accident**

In a life-threatening emergency a surgeon may act in what they consider to be the best interests of the patient. In this situation blood is usually given as part of emergency resuscitation, unless the patient has already told medical staff that they do not wish to have a transfusion (such as Jehovah's Witness). The risk of transmitting HIV infection from a unit of blood is approximately 1 in 106. Although patients are generally being ventilated well before decisions need to be made about organ donation this is not a problem. The issue here is that even if the patient has a donor card, the permission of the relatives must be obtained before organ donation is offered. Unless an investigation is relevant to the immediate management of the patient it should not be performed. Only if the surgeon had evidence of serious criminal or dangerous antisocial behaviour would it be acceptable to consider breach of confidentiality and disclose such information to the police.

5.82 Obtaining informed consent   Answers: AB

A moral right is one which it is generally accepted an individual can claim over others, who must respect it regardless of their own wishes. Autonomy allows for an individual's right to self determination including their right to determine their medical future. It is also necessary to attempt to ensure that a patient really understands the information that has been given to them before it can be considered that informed consent has been obtained when they sign a form. Even if a patient is detained for psychiatric treatment they may be capable of understanding and giving or withholding consent to a surgical procedure. Only if they are considered mentally incapable of this can the surgeon together with their psychiatric team make a decision which they consider to be in the patient's best interests. Whilst the views of children should be considered and treated with respect it is accepted that in many cases they may not be making a properly considered decision. It is for their parents or guardian to consent to or refuse treatment. Only when the surgeon considers that the parents or guardian may not be acting in the child's best interests may this be contested.

5.83 Patient confidentiality   Answers: ADE

With the exceptions of judicial requests, notifiable diseases, NHS investigations/tribunals and suspected terrorist activities all disclosures of confidential information are discretionary. In the case of criminal activities and dangerous antisocial behaviour the surgeon must have evidence, not merely suspicions, before contemplating a breach of confidentiality.

INDEX

Numbers given refer to the relevant question number. The word shown may not always be used in the question, but may appear in the explanatory answer.

Index

Index

Index

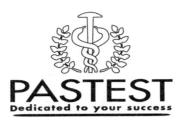